Chiropractic, Health Promotion, and Wellness

Meridel I. Gatterman, MA, DC, Med

Chair of the American Chiropractic Association
Subcommittee on Wellness Education

with contributions by

Ron Kirk, MA, DC

JONES AND BARTLETT PUBLISHERS
Sudbury, Massachusetts
BOSTON   TORONTO   LONDON   SINGAPORE

World Headquarters
Jones and Bartlett Publishers
40 Tall Pine Drive
Sudbury, MA 01776
978-443-5000
info@jbpub.com
www.jbpub.com

Jones and Bartlett Publishers Canada
6339 Ormindale Way
Mississauga, Ontario L5V 1J2
CANADA

Jones and Bartlett Publishers International
Barb House, Barb Mews
London W6 7PA
UK

Jones and Bartlett's books and products are available through most bookstores and online booksellers. To contact Jones and Bartlett Publishers directly, call 800-832-0034, fax 978-443-8000, or visit our website at www.jbpub.com.

Library of Congress Cataloging-in-Publication Data
Not available at time of publication.

6048

Production Credits
Executive Editor: David Cella
Editorial Assistant: Lisa Gordon
Production Director: Amy Rose
Production Editor: Renée Sekerak
Marketing Manager: Emily Ekle
Assistant Marketing Manager: Laura Kavigian
Manufacturing Buyer: Amy Bacus

Composition: Publishers Design and
    Production Services, Inc.
Cover Design: Kate Ternullo
Cover Image: © Photos.com
Printing and Binding: Malloy, Inc.
Cover Printing: Malloy, Inc.

Printed in the United States of America
10 09 08 07 06   10 9 8 7 6 5 4 3 2 1

This book is dedicated to patients who seek wellness through a partnership with doctors of chiropractic.

Contents

Foreword

A ccording to the actuaries at the Centers for Medicare and Medicaid Services, in 1970 the total expenditure on health care (public and private) in the United States was $73.1 billion. This amounted to 7% of the gross domestic product (GDP). This increased to $1.773 trillion, or 15.3% of the GDP, in 2004. Or, to look at it another way, the 2004 healthcare costs were 4.7 times that of the expenditure of the U.S. Department of Defense in fiscal year 2004, at the time of the war in Iraq. In 2000 the World Health Organization reported a health system performance assessment of the 191 member states of that organization. Of those 191 member countries, the United States ranked 72nd in its "efficiency of use" of healthcare resources.

So who pays the bills for all of this health care? We do—you and I. We pay them either through our taxes, our employee benefits, our insurance coverage, or out of our own pockets. And that is appropriate, since it is our own health and wellness that we are paying for.

By now, you are probably scratching your head and wondering how we can stop, or at least slow, this runaway inflation of healthcare expenses. The answer is that the responsibility for controlling the accelerating costs of health care lies with each of us who is individually responsible for maintaining his or her own health. If each of us could spend just a little time each day focused on our own health, including monitoring our diet, getting some exercise, managing our stress, working on our posture, avoiding bad health habits, and so on, there would be an immediate and significant impact on the efficient use of our healthcare resources.

So how do we as individuals get involved in a program that allows us to learn about and perform these health promotion activities to create a better state of health? That, my friend, is exactly what this book is about. Dr. Gatterman has tried to lay out the road map for each of us, as healthcare consumers, to follow in our pursuit of health and wellness. This book will walk you through health screening, nutrition, fitness, health promotion, and many other aspects of performance enhancement that, along with support from your doctor of chiropractic, can assist you in arriving at a more optimal state of health. Dr. Kirk has provided a chapter on spinal health, and Appendix A provides a quick and practical set of exercises to support a healthy spine. If there ever was an "owner's manual" for the human body, this is it! I hope you enjoy reading and learning about how to become a healthier you.

George B. McClelland, DC

Traditionally, doctors of chiropractic have promoted health and wellness by counseling patients on healthy lifestyles. Although chiropractors are best known for skilled manual therapy, the patient-centered nature of chiropractic care has been fundamental to chiropractic practice. This book explains how doctors of chiropractic work as partners with patients to promote health and wellness. Their approach to the whole patient emphasizes self-healing and conservative care.

Chapter 1 explores the chiropractic wellness model. The qualifications of doctors of chiropractic are discussed in Chapter 2. Identifying risky behavior that compromises health and prevents wellness is explored in Chapter 3. The contributions of mental and physical fitness to health and wellness are the subjects of Chapter 4. Nutritional guidelines are presented in Chapter 5 because "you are what you eat." Chapter 6 discusses the chiropractor's role in promoting spinal health and the contribution of the spine to health and well-being. Chapter 7 presents ways that you can reach optimal performance both at work and play. The final chapter describes ways that you can find a certified chiropractic wellness doctor to guide you in becoming healthier.

Doctors of chiropractic play an important role as health educators. They promote health and wellness in patients by working as partners in the evaluation and management of lifestyles and attitudes that can be changed. Health and wellness are not promoted by a disease-based healthcare system. A patient-centered model that provides individualized care can promote your health and well-being.

Acknowledgments

I am grateful to Dr. Ron Kirk for contributing the chapter on spinal health promotion and for his initiation and facilitation of the Straighten Up America program. I appreciate the generative contribution of the American Chiropractic Association Wellness Core Committee chaired by Dr. Ron Rupert under the direction of Dr. George McClelland. Appreciation is also expressed to Dr. Cheryl Hawk for reviewing the manuscript and making editorial comments.

Gratitude is expressed to the staff of Jones and Bartlett for assistance in bringing the book to production, including David Cella, executive editor; Jack Bruggeman, executive editor; Lisa Gordon, editorial assistant; Katilyn Crowley, editorial assistant; and Cara Judd for the illustrations.

Finally, my love and appreciation go to my husband, Mike Jamison, for insisting that I undertake this book, and for his continued support, understanding, and patience during its completion.

Chapter 1

The Chiropractic Wellness Model

The greatest of follies is to sacrifice health for any other advantage.

Schopenhauer

Doctors of chiropractic have traditionally been wellness doctors by promoting the health of their patients. This has taken the form of counseling on habits and lifestyle.[1] The first book to describe standards of chiropractic practice noted that "chiropractic educational institutions place great emphasis on patient counseling."[2]

Without individual responsibility, wellness is not possible. Patients, while becoming increasingly well informed about health issues, cannot be held solely responsible for healthy lifestyles. Guidance and encouragement from trained health educators are important components of the health promotion and wellness equation. An individualistic approach that promotes your health requires a practitioner who serves as a health educator, is patient centered and well informed about wellness practices, and emphasizes conservative health care. Doctors of chiropractic thus facilitate wellness through determining your general state of health and then educating and encouraging you to follow healthy habits and a wellness lifestyle.

What Is Wellness?

Wellness is a way of life. It is a process of optimal functioning and creative adaptation involving all aspects of your life. It is an enjoyable approach to living that emphasizes the importance of achieving harmony in all aspects of your mind, body, and spirit. It is a lifestyle that creates the greatest potential for personal well-being. More than an absence of illness, it is a dynamic balance among all aspects of your person. It is an active process in which you pursue activities with the aim of achieving optimal functioning that promotes your health.[3]

The Characteristics of Patient-Centered Care

Although doctors of chiropractic are not the only clinicians who practice patient-centered care, this approach to patients is typical of chiropractic practice (Table 1.1).[4] Patient-centered practice emphasizes self-healing, a holistic approach to the patient, and a humanistic attitude regarding the patient/doctor partnership. Doctors of chiropractic who emphasize wellness in their practices work with you as a partner, preferring minimally invasive procedures and therapies. Chiropractors thus facilitate wellness by determining your general state of health and then using education and encouragement to change your habits and lifestyle for the better.

Self-Healing

Doctors of chiropractic have traditionally emphasized the innate ability of the body to heal. They have a detailed knowledge of the mechanisms that regulate and repair the human body (homeostasis). They promote a vital dynamic balance and emphasize the importance of a healthy immune system in the promotion of wellness. The goal of care is to optimize the interaction between the nervous system that controls all other body functions and the body's structural components, primarily the spine and supporting muscles and soft tissues. It is important to recognize that improvements in your health are not always attributable to a doctor's skill or treatment intervention. A cut can heal without the Band-Aid.

Table 1.1 *Characteristics of Patient-Centered Care*

1. Recognition and facilitation of the innate organization and adaptation of the person
2. Recognition that care should ideally focus on the total person
3. Acknowledgment and respect for the patient's values, beliefs, expectations, and healthcare needs
4. Promotion of the patient's health through a preference for drugless, minimally invasive, and conservative care
5. A proactive approach that encourages patients to take responsibility for their health
6. A partnership between the patient and patient-centered practitioner in decision making, emphasizing clinically effective and economically appropriate care based on various levels of evidence

Adapted from Gatterman MI. A patient-centered paradigm: a model for chiropractic education and research. *J Altern Complement Med.* 1995;1:371–386.

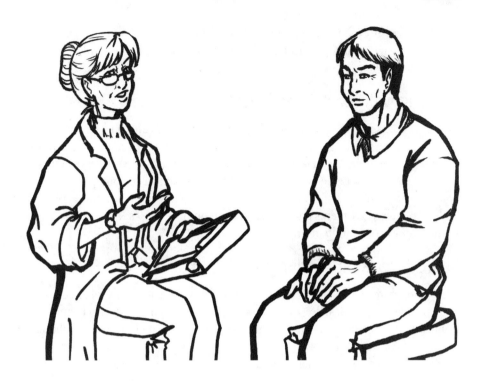

Holistic Health Care

Humans are complex organisms, and the causes of negative health events are multifactorial. A holistic approach to health care recognizes that there is a relationship among the component parts of your body. It is important that a diseased or dysfunctional body part not be seen as separate from your body as a whole. Wellness practitioners recognize that to achieve optimum health, doctors must treat the whole patient and not just diseases of isolated body parts. Care of the total person requires a willingness to address the full range of difficulties that you bring to your doctor, including psychological and social problems in addition to the physical dysfunctions that are customarily addressed.

A Humanistic Attitude

It is important that wellness practitioners acknowledge and respect your values, beliefs, healthcare needs, and expectations. They should approach you with unconditional positive regard, empathy, and genuineness. It is also important that they connect with you in meaningful and helpful ways. Doctors of chiropractic use physical contact to allay your fears, to establish therapeutic bonds, and to provide comfort.

Working with Patients as Partners

Wellness practitioners collaborate with you to promote health and facilitate wellness rather than needing to take charge of the process. They promote an active approach that encourages you to act responsibly for your health. Wellness doctors of chiropractic work together with you to develop a practical lifelong plan that encourages a healthy lifestyle. They invest time and energy to incorporate screening tools into their assessments and to counsel you on health risks, conservative interventions, and community resources.

Shared Decision Making

Doctors of chiropractic emphasize the importance of the patient's role in compliance with a healthy lifestyle. They work with you to manage effectively and economically the full range of your healthcare conditions, including those that are preventable or treatable and those that require referral to other practitioners. Chiropractic wellness practitioners have a logical set of beliefs based on scientific evidence that appeal to common sense, and they promote a holistic approach to health that facilitates wellness.[4]

Wellness: A Multidimensional Concept

Wellness is a multidimensional concept that includes physical, mental, spiritual, emotional, social, and environmental areas.[2] The traditional approach to health focuses primarily on the physical aspect of health. The doctor of chiropractic approaches your physical health by relating structure and function and by improving the modulating effect of the nervous system that enhances the body's natural recuperative ability.

Mental fitness is enhanced through health-promoting decision making and cognitive changes that make you better able to cope with daily stresses. Empowering you to take control of situations reduces the feelings of helplessness that have negative effects on your immune system. Spiritual health is related to having a sense of value and recognition of your life purpose. Spiritual well-being is encouraged through creative development and care of the self. Emotional health is related to self-esteem, self-efficacy, trust, and the ability to express emotions appropriately. Emotional coping skills that develop self-support and self-affirmation can replace "self-downing" through encouragement and counseling.

Social support and healthy interpersonal relationships are important to your wellness. Social isolation is a health risk, whereas building a good social support system mobilizes healing forces. Environmental factors contribute significantly to overall wellness. A sense of appreciation and responsibility for your relationship to the environment can significantly improve your health and environmental quality.

Accurate current information is a prerequisite for making informed decisions. Doctors of chiropractic can guide you in decision making that promotes health and facilitates wellness. They are trained to consider the multidimensional factors that contribute to your optimal well-being.

Understanding and Improving Health

Areas where doctors of chiropractic can help patients to understand the factors that improve health include wellness promotion, nutrition counseling, healthy activities of daily living, and occupational factors related to health.

- *Wellness promotion:* Doctors of chiropractic evaluate you for leading health indicators. These include tobacco use, substance abuse, responsible sexual behavior, injury and violence, immunization, and access to health care. Through screening and risk assessment your individual needs are determined. Counseling for lifestyle modification is also tailored to you as an individual. A partnership for promoting wellness can then be developed that may include health contracts based on a practical plan for achieving wellness. Depending on each patient's lifestyle plan, injury prevention can also be determined.

- *Nutrition:* Optimal nutrition is also an individual factor affecting health, based on needs, preferences, and availability (see Chapter 5). Doctors of chiropractic promote the essentials for healthy eating and minimal requirements for a healthy diet and discuss food for health. Food sensitivities and allergies are also considered. Body mass index and factors that contribute to a healthy weight are assessed. Weight problems, including underweight, overweight, and obesity, and eating disorders are addressed.

- *Activities:* Doctors of chiropractic are specialists in posture and spinal health and offer evaluation and correction of factors in these areas that affect wellness (see Chapter 6). They also assess your sleep, rest, and recreation patterns, which contribute to overall health. Stress management is recommended where needed. A program of physical activity and exercise is individualized to your needs for maximum effectiveness. Counseling regarding factors that promote mental fitness and reduce psychosocial stressors is also offered (see Chapter 4).

- *Occupational health:* Health factors related to work safety, in addition to the treatment and rehabilitation of on-the-job injuries, are important components of chiropractic practice. Environmental quality significantly affects health and preventable illnesses. The effects of a destructive environment are addressed. Workplace efficiency can be enhanced through screening and assessment of posture and movement associated with job tasks. Adjustment of work areas for greater safety and efficiency significantly prevents injury from trauma and microtrauma (see Chapter 7).

Individualizing Your Wellness Program

The doctor of chiropractic must first help you to develop a clear understanding and personal definition of health. The questions "What is *health*?" and "What does optimal health and wellness mean to you?" should be answered. A current personal health status assessment is the next step. Areas of weakness in your current health care can be established by means of questionnaires and health screening tools. A disease risk assessment is also important. Knowledge of the disorders to which you are most prone provides a specific direction for your health promotion focus. Delineation and ranking of your personal health goals should follow your personal health assessment. This is the starting point from which a rational, individualized healthcare program can be developed. After listing your goals, these should be discussed with your doctor of chiropractic, who may want to suggest some changes to your priority listing. Working as partners, agreement on health goals can be reached.

You can then begin to develop strategies for attaining your stated health goals. The resources of the healthcare system combined with your personal knowledge and skills can minimize your risk of disease and enhance your opportunity for wellness. The health plan you develop can be modified to suit your habits and preferences. Selected strategies can then be implemented based on the strategies decided upon, utilizing a personalized health management contract. Any difficulties encountered should be discussed with your doctor of chiropractic. If the program is too strenuous or unrealistic, changes to the contract can be made, using more realistic intermediary goals. Ongoing self-evaluation is a method of monitoring your progress. Continual feedback is essential as a health dynamic, and your practitioner should help you formulate a practical monitoring system.[5]

Health promotion, disease prevention, and wellness are appropriate challenges for all persons regardless of age. The achievement of optimal health and wellness enhances the enjoyment of life. The avoidance of disease prevents suffering and loss of productivity. Your optimal health and wellness is the best health deal you can make at any point in time.[5]

What Makes Doctors of Chiropractic Suitable as Wellness Clinicians?

Doctors of chiropractic are specialists in the treatment of conditions that affect the musculoskeletal system. These common disorders are best treated by conservative methods before they become chronic and require more invasive intervention such as drugs and surgery. Doctors of chiropractic also understand the relationship between the mind and the body and the nature of functional conditions that respond to conservative care.

Doctors of chiropractic are able to aid you in decisions affecting individual wellness because they are readily accessible. Chiropractic offices are located in most communities and provide easy access to chiropractic services. Doctors of chiropractic are primary contact practitioners and may serve as primary care doctors, making them ideally suited to solve health problems. They offer conservative care with a preference for natural, minimally invasive, and drugless interventions. They are committed to promoting health and they facilitate wellness by considering the many factors that contribute to your well-being.

References

1. Christensen MG, Kerkhooff D, Kollasch MW. *Analysis of Chiropractic*. Greeley, CO: National Board of Chiropractic Examiners; 2000.

2. Vear HJ. *Chiropractic Standards of Practice and Quality Care*. Gaithersburg, MD: Aspen; 1992:49–61.

3. Hawk C. Wellness hypothesis. In: Leach R, ed. *The Chiropractic Theories: A Textbook of Scientific Research*. Baltimore: Lippincott Williams & Wilkins; 2004:399–416.

4. Gatterman MI. A patient-centered paradigm: a model for chiropractic education and research. *J Altern Complement Med*. 1995;1:371–386.

5. Jamison JR. *Health Promotion for Chiropractic Practice*. Gaithersburg, MD: Aspen; 1991:29.

Chapter 2

Chiropractic Training in Health Promotion and Wellness Care

Chiropractors, now included as members of the orthodox health care system, work at the consumer-health system interface.

Jennifer Jamison

Chiropractors as Primary Contact Practitioners

As primary contact practitioners, chiropractors share the responsibility of licensed health professionals for promoting health and preventing disease.[1]

Licensure

By law, licensed chiropractors are entitled to use the titles "Doctor of Chiropractic" or "Chiropractic Physician." Chiropractors are licensed in all 50 states in the United States and all 10 provinces in Canada. The practice of chiropractic has continued to spread worldwide in the past two decades. Chiropractors promote health and wellness in addition to engaging in the treatment and prevention of disease. In North America, stringent educational and competency standards must be met before chiropractors can become licensed.

The Federation of Chiropractic Licensing Boards

In North America, chiropractic licensure is regulated by state and provincial licensing boards. The Federation of Chiropractic Licensing Boards (FCLB) maintains a directory of state-mandated requirements and procedures. The scope of practice varies from one jurisdiction to another. The FCLB was formed in 1993 to promote unified standards for chiropractic licensing boards and colleges. The FCLB provides a forum for state licensing board members to meet and address common areas of interest and concern. In addition, the FCLB maintains a computerized record of chiropractic licensure violations and disciplinary actions nationwide.

Education

Four steps must be followed before the doctor of chiropractic can practice (Table 2.1). The training of chiropractors includes two to four years of college prior to entering an accredited chiropractic college.[1] Minimum prerequisites include science and humanities credits (Table 2.2). Programs that graduate doctors of

Table 2.1 *Steps Leading to Chiropractic Practice*

1. Complete required general college-level studies (bachelor's degree required by some states).
2. Obtain a Doctor of Chiropractic degree and complete clinical externship through accredited four-year chiropractic college program.
3. Pass the National Board of Chiropractic Examiners' and/or other state-required examinations.
4. Satisfy any other individual state's specific requirements for licensure.

Reprinted with permission from Christensen MG. *Job Analysis of Chiropractic. A Project Report, Survey Analysis, and Summary of the Practice of Chiropractic within the United States*. Greeley, CO: National Board of Chiropractic Examiners; 2005.

Table 2.2 *Required Minimum Prerequisites*

Communication and/or language skills	6 semester hours
Psychology	3 semester hours
Social sciences or humanities	15 semester hours
Biological sciences with laboratory	6 semester hours
General or inorganic chemistry with laboratory	6 semester hours
Organic chemistry with laboratory	6 semester hours
Physics with laboratory	6 semester hours

Reprinted with permission from Christensen MG. *Job Analysis of Chiropractic. A Project Report, Survey Analysis, and Summary of the Practice of Chiropractic within the United States*. Greeley, CO: National Board of Chiropractic Examiners; 2005.

chiropractic are four to five years in length. The training for a Doctor of Chiropractic degree requires a minimum of six years of college study and an externship prior to entering private practice.[2] The typical chiropractic curriculum is outlined in Table 2.3.[1] Government inquiries, as well as independent investigations by medical practitioners, have affirmed that today's chiropractic training is of equivalent standard to medical training in preclinical subjects.[2] Clinical training is similar to that taught in medical schools, with an emphasis on conservative care, especially manual skills, instead of drugs and surgery.[3]

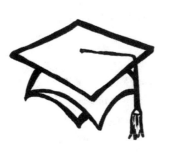
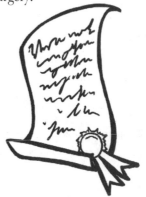

Chiropractic Undergraduate Courses That Promote Health and Wellness

The doctor of chiropractic is required to take courses that provide a basis for the understanding of nutrition. These include the biochemistry of proteins, enzymes, carbohydrates, lipids, vitamins, and trace elements. Clinical nutrition courses discuss nutrient metabolism and nutritional needs throughout life. Nutritional management of common conditions encountered in chiropractic practice is emphasized. Pediatric, maternal and infant, and geriatric courses discuss the specific needs of these different age groups.

Public health information is included for leading health indicators (tobacco use, substance abuse, responsible sexual behavior, injury and violence, immunization, and access to health care). Training in screening and risk assessment, along with counseling for lifestyle modification and injury prevention, is included. A patient-centered partnership for promoting wellness is an important part of traditional chiropractic care.

The strong emphasis on the neuromusculoskeletal system provides a background in the assessment and management of patients' posture and spinal health. Enhancement of function through physical activity and exercise is approached, considering individual variations and needs. Occupational health is considered in

Table 2.3 *Typical Chiropractic Curriculum*

First-year coursework

General anatomy	Human biochemistry
Histology	Clinical chiropractic
Palpation	Normal radiographic anatomy
Human physiology	Fundamentals of nutrition
Chiropractic procedures	Functional anatomy/biomechanics
Embryology	Spinal anatomy
Introduction to physical exam skills	Neuroanatomy and neurophysiology
Chiropractic principles	

Second-year coursework

Pharmatoxicology	Clinical Microbiology
Pathology	Chiropractic principles
Chiropractic procedures	Physics and clinical imaging
Clinical orthopedics and neurology	Nutritional assessment
Community/public health	Physiological therapeutics
Clinical nutrition	Research methods
Practice management	Imaging interpretation
Differential diagnosis	Applied clinical chiropractic
Emergency care	

Third-year coursework

Chiropractic clinical application	Physiological therapeutics
Chiropractic principles	Practice management
Radiological positioning and technique	Imaging interpretation
Application of manual procedures	Differential diagnosis
Clinical internship	Dermatology
Clinical psychology	Obstetrics /gynecology
Pediatrics	Geriatrics
Clinical laboratory clerkship	Ethics and jurisprudence
Original research project	

Fourth-year

Clinical internship

The Doctor of Chiropractic (D.C.) is awarded upon graduation, signifying successful completion of the required program.

Reprinted with permission from Christensen MG. *Job Analysis of Chiropractic. A Project Report, Survey Analysis, and Summary of the Practice of Chiropractic within the United States*. Greeley, CO: National Board of Chiropractic Examiners; 2005.

terms of work safety, environmental quality, and ergonomics. Mental fitness that is dependent on sleep, rest, and recreation in addition to stress management is discussed relative to individual patient needs.

Although chiropractic undergraduate programs provide instruction in counseling that encourages healthful living practices and wellness procedures, some doctors of chiropractic seek additional training (see Chapter 8).[4] Nearly all doctors of chiropractic instruct patients regarding health promotion and wellness. Advice on general fitness and exercise promotion is given by over 98% of chiropractors.[1]

Accreditation

The Council on Chiropractic Education (CCE), the accrediting body that sets the standards for chiropractic education, considers that doctors of chiropractic must be able to provide wellness care and to promote health maintenance as well as to perform common screening procedures and wellness assessments in different age groups.[5] The CCE also states that a doctor of chiropractic should be trained to help meet the health needs of individuals and of the public, including wellness promotion by assessing health risks and providing general health information and lifestyle counseling.[6]

Examinations

Part I of the standard exam set by the National Board of Chiropractic Examiners includes general anatomy, spinal anatomy, physiology, chemistry, pathology, microbiology, and public health.[7] Clinical subjects examined in Part II include general diagnosis, neuromuscular diagnosis, diagnostic imaging, principles of chiropractic, and associated clinical sciences. The associated clinical sciences include geriatrics, pediatrics, dermatology, emergency procedures, psychology, gynecology and obstetrics, and toxicology, as well as the study of sexually transmitted diseases and jurisprudence.

Part III emphasizes conservative drugless and noninvasive care, including the case history, physical examination, neuromusculoskeletal examination, the roentgenologic examination, clinical laboratory and special studies, diagnosis or clinical impression, chiropractic manual techniques, case management, and supportive techniques. Supportive techniques include physiotherapy, nutrition, corrective exercise, protective body mechanics (ergonomics), and patient education and home care.[7]

Prior to graduation, doctors of chiropractic participate in internship training at clinics similar to the typical chiropractic office.[2] This training provides a practical experience that prepares them to counsel patients in health promotion strategies that lead to wellness. Part IV of the national examination consists of a hands-on practical examination that ensures that graduating chiropractors are proficient in diagnostic imaging, chiropractic techniques, and case management.

Scope of Chiropractic Practice

Nearly all doctors of chiropractic instruct patients regarding health promotion and wellness. The Association of Chiropractic Colleges includes health promotion in its statement of the scope of chiropractic practice.[8] Advice on general fitness and exercise promotion is given by over 98% of chiropractors.[2] Over 90% of chiropractic physicians provide nutrition and dietary recommendations, ergonomic and postural advice, counseling on changing risky and unhealthy behaviors, self-care strategies, relaxation and stress recommendations, and disease prevention and early screening advice.[2] Not every patient receives health promotion and wellness counseling based on individual preferences and needs.

Specialization

Postdoctoral specialization training is available in a variety of disciplines and specialties through accredited chiropractic colleges. Some courses are offered through part-time postgraduate education programs, whereas others are full-time residency programs. Postgraduate specialty education programs are listed in Tables 2.4 and 2.5. Both postgraduate and residency programs lead to eligibility to sit for competency examinations recognized by the American Board of Chiropractic Specialties and the International Chiropractic Association. Specialty boards may confer "Diplomate" status in a given area of expertise upon successful

Table 2.4 *Postgraduate Education Programs*

Family practice	Applied chiropractic science
Clinical neurology	Orthopedics
Sports chiropractic	Pediatrics
Nutrition	Rehabilitation
Industrial counseling	Radiology
Integrative health and wellness	

Reprinted with permission from Christensen MG. *Job Analysis of Chiropractic. A Project Report, Survey Analysis, and Summary of the Practice of Chiropractic within the United States*. Greeley, CO: National Board of Chiropractic Examiners; 2005.

Table 2.5 *Chiropractic Residency Programs*

Radiology	Orthopedics
Family practice	Clinical sciences

examination. The most common specialty certification areas are chiropractic orthopedics, radiology, and sports chiropractic.[2]

The Clinical Dilemma of Health Care

Medicine has achieved some diminution in the uncertainty associated with disease pathology by using a reductionistic model. The science of clinical medicine is based on precise observations and theories of causation, decision making, and evidence.[1]

Basing clinical care on a disease model has enabled the observation and classification of a group of signs and symptoms into identifiable syndromes with somewhat predictable outcomes. This model is ideal for disease care but has little relevance to health care or health promotion. The clinical application of this model is *curing* rather than *caring*. The inadequacy of this model fails to encompass health promotion and wellness.[1]

The primary contact framework of chiropractic wellness care encompasses a holistic model that considers lifestyle and promotes health. Health is not merely the absence of disease. Health encompasses an active lifestyle that leads to wellness and optimal vitality. This approach to health care is based on interventions that include counseling and health education as their management strategies. Successful implementation of wellness care is based on a partnership between you and your chiropractor.

If you become a chiropractic patient seeking care for a health problem, you will want to discuss wellness care with your chiropractor. In other cases you may seek the services of a chiropractor who practices health promotion and wellness even though you do not have an identifiable health problem. Remember, wellness care can add significantly to your quality of life.

References

1. Jamison J. *Health Promotion for Chiropractic Practice*. Gaithersburg, MD: Aspen; 1991:167–172.

2. Christensen MG. *Job Analysis of Chiropractic. A Project Report, Survey Analysis, and Summary of the Practice of Chiropractic within the United States*. Greeley, CO: National Board of Chiropractic Examiners; 2005.

3. Chapman-Smith D. *Chiropractic: A Referenced Source of Modern Concepts*. Palmerton, PA: Practice Makers Products; 1988.

4. Hawk C, Rupert RL, Hyland JK, Odhwani A. Implementation of a course on wellness concepts into a chiropractic college curriculum. *J Manipulative Physiol Ther*. 2005;28(6):423–428.

5. Council on Chiropractic Education, Commission on Accreditation. *Standards for Doctor of Chiropractic Programs and Institutions*. Scottsdale, AZ: Council on Chiropractic Education; 2003.

6. Council on Chiropractic Education, Commission on Accreditation. *Standards for Doctor of Chiropractic Programs and Institutions*. Scottsdale, AZ: Council on Chiropractic Education; 2004.

7. National Board of Chiropractic Examiners. *NBCE Examination Information: Part I, Part II, Part III* [brochure]. Greeley, CO: National Board of Chiropractic Examiners; 2004.

8. Association of Chiropractic Colleges. *Chiropractic Scope of Practice Consensus Statement*. Bethesda, MD: Association of Chiropractic Colleges; July 1996. Position Paper 1.

Chapter 3

Identifying Risky Behavior

The nature of chiropractic care with its health-oriented philosophical basis is well positioned to influence patient attitudes about life style related health behaviors.

Alan Adams

Y ou have the ability to judge your own health status given adequate information. Safe self-assessment is only possible when you know when to seek a
professional opinion.[1] Wellness involves a personal health promotion program that includes screening for disease in addition to determining health status
on the disease–wellness continuum. Health and disease are not discrete entities,
but rather a relative state on a sliding scale (Figure 3.1).[1] Where you fall on this
continuum can be assessed by your doctor of chiropractic using screening procedures that can reduce risky behaviors that affect your health.[2]

Following the wellness model (Figure 3.2) potentially maximizes your full
health potential. Your greatest degree of well-being is achieved by health risk ap-
praisal, health fitness evaluation, and health promotion. Your doctor of chiropractic can help you to modify your lifestyle by serving as both your health
educator and health promotion manager.

Leading Health Indicators

Information about leading health indicators is an important first step in assessment of your health. Healthy People 2010 lists ten health indicators chosen
for their ability to motivate action (Table 3.1).[2] These health indicators include

Figure 3.1 *The Disease–Wellness Continuum*

Disease pole _____ **Wellness pole**

Figure 3.2 *The Wellness Model*

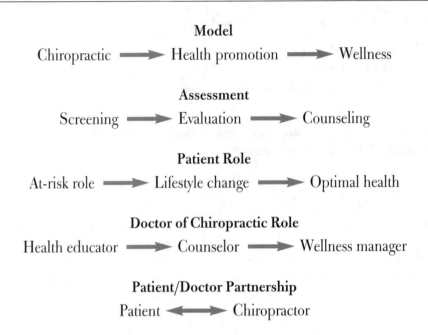

individual behaviors, such as physical, psychological, social, and environmental factors, and issues that affect your health. The process of selecting these indicators was led by an interagency work group within the U.S. Department of Health and Human Services. The leading health indicators are intended to help you more easily understand factors that lead to health promotion, disease prevention, and optimal wellness. Doctors of chiropractic can help you determine your health risks through noninvasive screening and develop strategies and action plans that address these health indicators so you can increase the quality of your life.

Table 3.1 *Leading Health Indicators*

Physical activity	Mental health
Overweight and obesity	Injury and violence
Tobacco use	Environmental quality
Substance abuse	Immunization
Responsible sexual behavior	Access to health care

Physical Activity

Regular physical activity throughout life is important for maintaining a healthy body and enhancing psychological well-being. Regular physical activity promotes a healthy heart, lowers the risk of developing diabetes, and is associated with a decreased risk of colon cancer.[2] Regular physical activity also helps to prevent and reduce high blood pressure in addition to aiding in weight control, increasing muscle and bone strength, and improving mental health.[2] Screening for physical fitness must consider individual differences. These include your current level of physical activity, individual needs and preferences, and available resources. Safety requirements include ruling out conditions that require professional supervision of individualized exercise programs (see Chapter 4).

Weight Control

Overweight and obesity substantially raise your risk of a variety of diseases. These include high blood pressure, diabetes, heart disease and stroke, gallbladder disease, arthritis, sleep disorders, breathing problems, and some types of cancer. Obese individuals also may suffer from social discrimination and lowered self-esteem.[2] A healthy diet (see Chapter 5) and regular physical activity (see Chapter 4) are both important for maintaining a healthy weight. Eating disorders that lead to falling below a healthy weight may be serious enough to be life threatening.

Measurement of your height to determine your ideal body weight from height and weight charts is a poor method of screening for weight disorders. Utilizing these charts may indicate too much weight if you have a heavy frame with a high proportion of muscle that weighs more than fat, or an acceptable weight if you have a small frame with a high proportion of fat that may be unhealthy. Screening for composition of body mass and energy requirements offers a positive method of weight control.[3] Determination of your energy intake will help you maintain ideal body weight.

Tobacco Use

Cigarette smoking is the single most preventable cause of disease and death in the United States. Smoking results in more deaths each year in the United States than AIDS, alcohol, cocaine, heroin, homicide, suicide, motor vehicle crashes, and fires combined. Smoking is a major risk factor for heart disease, stroke, lung cancer, and chronic lung diseases—all leading causes of death. Smoking during pregnancy can result in miscarriages, premature delivery, and sudden infant death syndrome. Fire-related injuries and environmental damage caused by fires are other effects of smoking. Secondhand smoke increases the risk of heart disease and significant lung conditions, especially asthma and bronchitis in children. There is no safe tobacco alternative to cigarettes. Spit tobacco (chew), cigars, and pipe smoking also increase the risk of cancer.[2] Although many health practitioners are pessimistic about their ability to persuade people to quit smoking, the doctor of chiropractic can enhance your ability to quit smoking if this is a consideration in your wellness program.[1]

Substance Abuse

Excessive use of alcohol and other recreational drugs is associated with serious health problems. The annual economic costs to the United States from alcohol abuse were estimated to be $167 billion in 1995. In 1998, 17% of adults aged 18 years and older when surveyed reported binge drinking in the past month, which was defined as consuming five or more drinks on one occasion. Alcohol abuse is associated with motor vehicle crashes, homicides, suicides, and drowning—leading causes of death among youth. Long-term heavy drinking can lead to heart disease, cancer, alcohol-related liver disease, and pancreatitis. Alcohol use during pregnancy is known to cause fetal alcohol syndrome, a leading cause of mental retardation.[2] Screening for warning signs of excessive use of alcohol is a useful device for people who are drinking too much and have failed to recognize the warning signs. Light alcohol consumption may be beneficial, and it has been suggested that there is less risk of coronary heart disease if you drink one alcoholic drink each day.[3]

Responsible Sexual Behavior

Sexually transmitted diseases (STDs) and unintended pregnancies can result from unprotected sexual behaviors. Abstinence is the only method of complete protection. Condoms can help prevent both STDs and unintended pregnancy if used correctly and consistently. Half of all pregnancies in the United States are unintended; that is, at the time of conception the pregnancy was not planned or not wanted. It is possible for you to become infected with an STD by a partner who has no symptoms.[2] If you are sexually active, you should know how to recognize the symptoms of infection. All sexually active persons should know how to practice safe sex. Screening for safe sex can tell you if you are at risk for STDs and unwanted pregnancies.

Mental Health

No one is immune to mental illness, and approximately 20% of the U.S. population is affected to some degree during a given year. Depression is the most common disorder. Major depression is a leading cause of disability and is the cause of more than two-thirds of suicides each year. Mental health is sometimes thought of as simply the absence of mental illness, but it is actually much broader. Mental health is a successful state of mental functioning, resulting in productive activities, fulfilling relationships, and the ability to adapt to change and cope with adversity.[2] Mental health is indispensable to your well-being, family and interpersonal relationships, and your contribution to society.

Depression can be recognized through screening, with different forms of treatment recommendations. Counseling and other conservative treatment for mild depression can be recommended by your doctor of chiropractic and referral made if other treatment is indicated. Strategies that enhance the coping skills that are a large part of wellness can be taught and learned. A sense of personal control can be developed that contributes significantly to mental fitness (see Chapter 4).[1]

Injury and Violence

The risk of injury is so great that most persons sustain a significant injury at some time during their lives. Motor vehicle crashes are the most common cause of serious injury. They are often predictable and preventable. Increased use of safety belts and reductions in driving while impaired are two of the most effective means to reduce the risk of death and serious injury of occupants in motor vehicle crashes.[2] A motor vehicle accident risk index can identify your risk of being injured in a motor vehicle accident. You can then modify your driving habits to lower your risk. Home safety can be increased when a checklist of factors that reduce the risk of accident in the home is identified. Recommendations for inexpensive equipment and modifications that increase your home safety can be made.[1]

Environmental Quality

Physical and social environments play major roles in your health and wellness. The physical environment includes the air, water, and soil, through which exposure to chemical, biological, and physical agents may occur. The social environment includes housing, transportation, urban development, industry, and agriculture and results in exposures such as work-related stress and injury.[2] Occupational activities and postures that pose risk factors for you can be identified, and safer and more efficient job design can reduce stress, fatigue, and injury. Screening and job analysis can lead to ergonomic structuring of the workplace by your doctor of chiropractic (see Chapter 7).

Immunization

Many once-common vaccine-preventable diseases are now controlled in the Western Hemisphere, including smallpox and poliomyelitis. The use of immunization should be restricted to increasing the individual's immunity to those diseases with significant mortality, morbidity, or economic consequences. Successful immunization requires that you have a healthy immune system in which a realistic biological challenge infection does not result in the clinical manifestation of the disease for which you have been immunized. Contraindications to the use of live vaccines include acute fevers, acute systemic viral infections, immune deficiency, corticosteroid or other immunosuppressant therapy, malignant disease, pregnancy, hypersensitivity to constituents of the vaccine, and passive immunity.

Complications attributable to immunization are considered to be far less frequent than those attributable to natural infections. The greatest risk has been associated with the pertussis (whooping cough) vaccine. Some of the most reported complications are attributable to the medium in which the vaccine is prepared. As with any healthcare procedure, it is important to consider the risks as well as benefits in order to give informed consent to that procedure.

Access to Health Care

Financial, structural, and personal barriers can limit access to health care. Financial barriers include not having health insurance, not having health insurance that covers needed services, or not having the financial capacity to cover health services outside a health plan or insurance program. Financial barriers are a serious consideration that must be addressed in this country since strong predictors of access to quality health care include having health insurance, a higher income level, and a regular primary care provider. It has been demonstrated that doctors of chiropractic as primary care providers in an integrative medicine organization provided care at substantially reduced costs for patients when compared with care given by medical doctors and osteopaths.[4]

Structural barriers include lack of primary care providers and access to healthcare facilities. Community-based chiropractic practices offer ready access to primary contact chiropractors in most areas.

Personal barriers include cultural or spiritual differences, language barriers, not knowing what to do or when to seek care, or concerns about confidentiality or discrimination. The patient-centered nature of chiropractic practice reduces personal barriers when care is individualized and your values, beliefs, and healthcare needs are respected.

Office Screening Procedures

Not all screening procedures for health promotion require expensive and invasive tests performed in laboratories or hospitals. Screening and information and counseling that promote wellness can be performed in the office of the doctor of chiropractic, including nutrition guidance, spinal hygiene, skeletal health promotion, healthy sleep, and hypertension. Screening for cholesterol levels, diabetes, osteoporosis, headaches, and back pain requires laboratory or radiographic imaging for adequate assessment. The doctor of chiropractic is qualified to screen for these conditions and is licensed to perform these services in most states.

Nutrition

Dietary guidelines should be periodically reviewed in the light of progress in nutritional sciences, changes in agricultural and food technologies, habits, health status, and socioeconomic situations. Government dietary recommendations endeavor to favorably modify eating habits and include recommended daily allowances (RDAs). RDAs are determined through research on laboratory animals and metabolic research on humans that provides information about energy and micronutrient requirements.

Individual variability mandates that your requirement for nutrients be assessed based on your genetic makeup, the availability of nutritious food, and your lifestyle. Dietary recommendations should be achievable through informed food choices and not solely through nutritional supplements.[3] Dietary advice must be based on assessment of individual requirements, with consideration of specific disorders that respond to modification of nutritional programs. Doctors of chiropractic are trained in the biochemistry of nutrition and can offer sound nutritional advice (see Chapter 5).

Spinal Health

Doctors of chiropractic have traditionally been known as proponents of spinal health. Good posture is fundamental to your spinal health and should be assumed when you are standing, lying, sitting, and bending. Good posture is not a static concept but involves changing positions and, more importantly, your everyday movements. The spine is the organ of posture and is a flexible column made up of 24 motion segments. Movement of these segments is essential to your spinal health, and misalignment or restricted movement (the chiropractic subluxation) leads to various forms of dysfunction. Screening for spinal health involves postural evaluation, and spinal palpation for misalignment and motion restriction. Doctors of chiropractic are specialists in the treatment of spinal motion segment dysfunction and postural distortion. Screening for scoliosis (spinal curvature) is an important part of a chiropractic physical examination. Spinal health is an important component of your state of wellness (see Chapter 6).[5]

Healthy Sleep, Rest, and Relaxation

Assessment of sleep patterns and habits of rest and relaxation is important to promote overall well-being. Sleep assessment may be made initially by maintaining a sleep diary.[3] A number of variables that predispose you to sleep disorders should be considered. If you are having difficulty with sleep, you may be helped by a sleep self-management program. When a conservative approach to sleep disorders fails, referral to a sleep center can be considered.[3] Inability to rest and relax can be assessed using an anxiety recognition chart.[3] Stress that contributes to the inability to relax can be managed conservatively by employing a number of self-care techniques after a variety of potential stressors have been identified (see Chapter 4).

High Blood Pressure (Hypertension)

High blood pressure is a disorder increasing with age and obesity. High blood pressure is listed as among the major risk factors for both stroke and heart disease. Regardless of age and weight, monitoring blood pressure is an important part of any wellness examination. Various factors can help you lower your blood pressure, if the condition is not severe. Restriction of salt, moderation in alcohol consumption, weight control, exercise, relaxation therapy, and chiropractic adjustments, especially to the thoracic spine, have all been helpful in lowering blood pressure. The side effects from drug therapy are undesirable, and a more conservative approach may be effective in less severe cases. Doctors of chiropractic can monitor your blood pressure in routine office visits, making referral for drug therapy when appropriate.

Muscle Pain and Fibromyalgia

Among the common conditions seen by doctors of chiropractic are those related to muscle pain, including fibromyalgia. Although rarely disabling, they can cause much needless suffering. Simple physical examination and palpatory tests can screen for these frequently misdiagnosed conditions. Treatment of muscle pain and fibromyalgia that focuses on a wellness program can significantly help you manage these conditions.[4]

Screening for Conditions That Require Special Tests

Not all screening can be done without special tests that require laboratory work or diagnostic imaging such as x-rays. Doctors of chiropractic are trained and licensed in most states to employ special tests for commonly seen conditions such as cholesterol levels, blood sugar (diabetes screening), and musculoskeletal pathology. Following spinal examination, x-rays may be required for common conditions seen by chiropractors, such as neck pain, headache, and back pain.

Cholesterol Screening

Monitoring unhealthy levels of cholesterol in the blood (hyperlipidemia) requires laboratory blood tests. Hyperlipidemia has been linked to heart disease and should be monitored in patients with a family member who has had a heart attack before the age of 55. Not all forms of cholesterol are harmful, and it is important that your screening differentiate between low-density lipoproteins and high-density lipoproteins (HDLs) and the total cholesterol to HDL ratio. Cholesterol levels can be affected by exercise and diet (see Chapters 4 and 5).

Diabetes

Diabetes is a common and serious condition; with its complications, it is the third most important cause of death attributable to disease in developed countries.[3] It is an important cause of blindness, diseases of blood circulation, neurological diseases, and kidney failure. The most convenient screening technique for diabetes is a simple blood test. Conservative management for diabetic control pivots around maintenance of an acceptable blood sugar level. Diet, exercise, and weight reduction are the main management goals in non-insulin-dependent diabetes. Drugs have an important role in the management of diabetes in severe cases, and drug therapy can be life saving. Care must be taken to balance insulin dose, food intake, exercise levels, and stress exposure.[3]

Osteoporosis

Skeletal health depends on production of adequate bone mass. Osteoporosis is a systemic disease characterized by a reduction in bone mass that results in increased susceptibility to fractures. If your screening questionnaire suggests the likelihood of future osteoporosis, then bone mass determination is in order. Ultrasound imaging of the heel is used to measure bone density at health fairs and in clinics. Dual-energy x-ray absorptiometry of the hip is considered the gold standard for predicting hip fracture from osteoporosis. Osteoporosis prevention is based on exercise and optimal nutrition early in life, adapted to your individual lifestyle and disease risk. Your doctor of chiropractic can assess your nutritional intake and exercise program, customizing both to your individual needs.

Neck Pain, Headache, and Back Pain

Doctors of chiropractic are specialists in the diagnosis and treatment of neck pain, headache, and back pain. Although diagnosing the cause of these common conditions may not require x-rays, they are frequently necessary to screen for nonmechanical causes. Experts in palpatory examinations, doctors of chiropractic use their hands to assess spinal function. Headaches caused by neck injuries from motor vehicle accidents and postural problems respond well to chiropractic care. In addition to manual therapies, an exercise program designed specifically for you can help reduce the pain and prevent recurrence.[4]

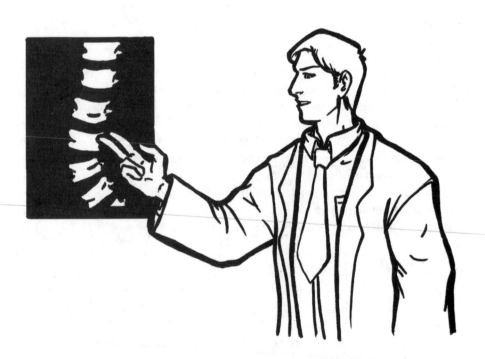

References

1. Jamison JR. *Maintaining Health in Primary Care: Guidelines for Wellness in the 21st Century*. St. Louis: Churchill Livingstone; 2001.

2. U.S. Department of Health and Human Services. *Healthy People 2010: Understanding and Improving Health*. 2nd ed. Washington, DC: U.S. Government Printing Office; November 2000.

3. Jamison JR. *Health Promotion for Chiropractic Practice*. Gaithersburg, MD: Aspen; 1991.

4. Sarnat RL, Winterstein J. Clinical and cost outcomes of an integrative medicine IPA. *J Manipulative Physiol Ther*. 2000;27:336–347.

5. Gatterman MI. *Chiropractic Management of Spine Related Disorders*. 2nd ed. Baltimore: Lippincott Williams & Wilkins; 2004.

Chapter 4

Mental and Physical Fitness

Since the time of the ancient Greeks, we have felt that there was a close relationship between a strong vital mind and physiological fitness.

John F. Kennedy

When we think of fitness, we frequently focus on physical fitness, yet mental fitness is also an important component of wellness. Your doctor of chiropractic can assess and guide you to maximize both the mental and physical fitness essential to achieving wellness. Your personal fitness can be achieved and maintained by working in a partnership with your chiropractor to design activities that lead to wellness.

Mental Fitness

Mental fitness is a state of successful mental functioning, resulting in productive activities, fulfilling relationships, and the ability to adapt to change and cope with adversity.[1] Mental fitness is indispensable to your personal well-being. It affects family and interpersonal relationships and your ability to contribute to society.[1]

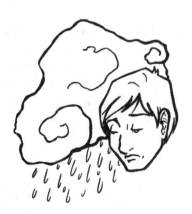 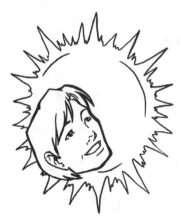

Strategies that enhance coping skills are a large part of mental fitness and can be taught and learned. A sense of personal control can be developed that contributes significantly to your mental fitness. Mental fitness is related to successful stress management. The ability to control stress both psychologically and neurochemically is a critical variable in your stress management and is emphasized in chiropractic wellness care.[2]

Assessment of Psychosocial Stressors

The assessment of psychosocial stressors can be accomplished by your doctor of chiropractic through a history of your family and home life, occupational and recreational life, spiritual and community life, and financial situation.[2] In addition, a rating scale that assesses life events for the previous year can determine your level of accumulated stress.[3] The importance of life events, your response to them, and the impact on your overall well-being can then be determined. The response of the autonomic nervous system to excessive stress over time leads to an imbalance between the sympathetic and parasympathetic nervous systems that can be addressed by doctors of chiropractic.[2]

ANGER AS A STRESSOR

Unresolved anger significantly affects your health and well-being. Negative anger results in hostility and is self-destructive when aggressive impulses are turned inward. Anger turned inward can increase your personal stress and lead to depression. When severe, unresolved anger can be addressed by referral for anger management. Coping with stress is a life skill. Dealing with angry people is another potential source of stress. Listening to what the other person is trying to convey rather than responding can often defuse the situation.[4]

PAIN AS A STRESSOR

Poorly controlled pain leads to mental as well as physical changes that severely compromise mental well-being. Central sensitization that magnifies chronic pain can result in conditions such as fibromyalgia and irritable bowel syndrome that can be treated by chiropractic care. Psychological distress from chronic pain may manifest as depression or apathy. Psychic pain can lead to self-medication with alcohol or drugs that then becomes a problem in itself.

Psychosomatic Syndromes

Psychosomatic syndromes have often been dismissed as being "just in your head." The mind–body connection has become better understood in the past 20 years.

The holistic approach of chiropractic wellness doctors acknowledges and addresses this connection.

Psychosomatic disorders can affect a number of different organ systems:[2]

- The respiratory system by triggering hyperventilation syndrome, chronic bronchitis, or asthma
- The cardiovascular system with high blood pressure, migraine headaches, or irregular heartbeats
- The gastrointestinal system with aggravation of peptic ulceration, irritable bowel syndrome, or anorexia nervosa
- The genitourinary system with menstrual disorders or frequent infections
- The musculoskeletal system with backache, neck pain, or tension headaches

Your doctor of chiropractic may recommend particular treatment for specific target organs in addition to stress management strategies that address the psychological component that is perpetuating the organ dysfunction.

Sleep Disorders

Acute stress and environmental disturbances can cause transient and short-term insomnia. More problematic is chronic insomnia that can develop in response to physical or psychosocial stressors. Sleep assessment may begin with a sleep diary. Factors that can affect your sleep habits include psychological stress, physical problems, shift work, jet lag, restless leg syndrome, excessive intake of caffeine, and compromised breathing (sleep apnea). Poorly controlled pain can prevent you from falling asleep and in turn wake you once you are asleep.

Narcolepsy is a chronic sleep disorder that produces severe problems with sleepiness. This can be as distressing as insomnia. Severe sleepiness can cause impairment comparable to that caused by alcohol intoxication. Both your sleep patterns and causes of your sleep disturbance must be assessed to successfully formulate your personal sleep regimen.

Stress Management

A holistic approach to stress management includes the following:[2]

- Regular relaxation sessions. Techniques such as meditation, visualization, tension release, or progressive muscular relaxation may be recommended.
- Regular exercise. An individualized exercise program can be designed to reduce stress and improve mental fitness.
- Outdoor activities that put you in contact with nature. Gardening or spending time in a beautiful park can be inexpensive ways of reducing stress.

- Sound nutrition. Excess alcohol and caffeine consumption should be avoided.
- Cessation of smoking or other forms of tobacco use.
- A balance between work and play. A realistic recreational program based on age, temperament, and level of physical fitness can be recommended for you.

Time Management

Efficient use of time depends on prioritization of daily tasks and life goals. Time can be wasted as a result of unnecessary personal behaviors adding to mental stress. Beware of the following:[4]

- *Perfectionism:* Setting unrealistic standards challenges perfectionistic tendencies.
- *Confusion:* Understand why you are performing a task; know your goals.
- *Indecision:* Decide how best to reach your desired goals.
- *Overload:* Do not attempt to do too much in the time available.
- *Procrastination:* Leaving it for later can become habitual.
- *Avoidance:* Do not put off a task so that it will go away.
- *Interruptions:* Distractions can prolong your tasks.
- *Being unable to say no:* By saying yes to one task, you are really saying no to something else, so be sure that you make the right choice.

Refining Coping Skills

Wellness promotion needs to be tailored specifically to your needs. Your commitment to lifestyle changes that promote mental fitness is a prerequisite to your successful wellness program. Mental fitness can be enhanced by refining coping skills. Referral for cognitive therapy can be effective in relieving depression and underlying anger. Cognitive therapy works to change thought patterns and can help you deal with difficult situations in specific realistic terms.[5] Changing your perspective of yourself and your attitudes toward others can have a dramatic effect that improves mental fitness.

Physical Fitness

Physical fitness, like mental fitness, promotes wellness. Physical inactivity is increasingly being recognized as a substantial health risk. Regular exercise retards the decline in physiological parameters characteristically associated with aging. Regular exercise can reduce degenerative diseases as well as slow the aging process and

increase your ability to meet emergencies. Your physical fitness may be achieved and maintained by continuing adherence to an appropriate exercise program.[2]

The most significant aspect of your physical fitness program is that it be tailored to your specific needs. Finding activities that are enjoyable; suit your age, gender, and body build; and are based on your individual needs contributes to a realistic exercise program. Your chiropractor understands that people with different body types find different physical activities enjoyable.[5] Tall, slender individuals tend to enjoy and excel at solitary activities such as running or jogging, swimming, and back country skiing. Stocky, heavily muscled individuals often have a high need for activity and enjoy contact sports and competitive cross-country skiing. If you are shorter and less muscular, you may enjoy more social activities and be drawn to activities such as bowling or volleyball. Body types may be used to guide you in the choice of physical activities, within limits. The form of exercise that best suits you is the only activity that is likely to be pursued regularly. Your doctor of chiropractic can guide and teach you to work toward optimal physical fitness through a practical exercise program.

Components of Physical Fitness

Physical fitness provides resistance to disease. Exercise is a planned, structured, and repetitive bodily movement that improves or maintains one or more components of physical fitness.[4] Physical fitness encompasses cardiovascular fitness, muscle strength and endurance, flexibility, balance, and body composition.

CARDIORESPIRATORY FITNESS

Exercise can improve your coronary artery blood flow, reduce heart muscle oxygen consumption, and increase your heart output.[2] A decrease in your blood pressure when slightly elevated can be achieved through adherence to a regular exercise program. It has been suggested that exercise may decrease your risk of heart attack. Exercise also increases your respiratory efficiency. Achievement of cardiorespiratory fitness requires aerobic exercise involving use of your large muscle groups. Activities such as swimming, cycling, walking, and running can produce cardiorespiratory fitness when done regularly. Only regular exercise energetically performed can influence cardiorespiratory fitness, and your exercise program should be designed to meet your individual needs.

MUSCLE STRENGTH AND ENDURANCE

Muscle strength is your capacity to tolerate workloads. Muscle strength is increased when you apply effort against resistance. Light resistance and increased

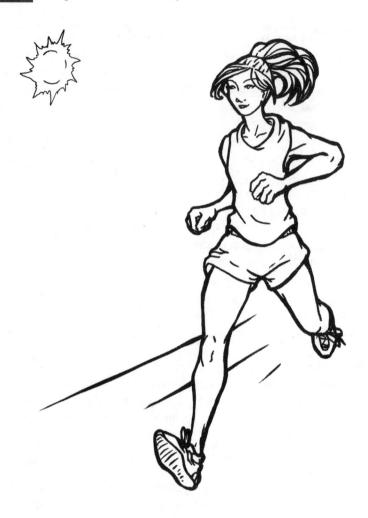

repetitions can increase your strength and tone your muscles without significant muscle building. You need enough strength to perform your daily tasks plus some extra to delay fatigue and prevent injury. Muscle endurance enables you to persist in an activity over a period of time. Building muscle strength and endurance to achieve wellness requires a gradual exercise program to prevent musculoskeletal injuries. Exercise planning ranges from selecting the right activity to meet your needs to selecting the appropriate equipment, including choosing the right shoes.

FLEXIBILITY

Flexibility is the component of fitness that maintains joint range of motion and optimal muscle length. Flexibility is joint specific and is best maintained through performing stretching exercises daily. You should hold stretching movements at the point of tightness, without proceeding to the point of pain. "No pain, no gain" should be replaced by the motto "train, don't strain."[2] When you participate regularly in exercise adapted to your needs and thereby attain a state of physical fitness, you may be called trained. Excessive joint movement can be as problematic as too little flexibility, especially if you do not maintain adequate strength to protect the joint from injury.

BALANCE

Balance is the maintenance of equilibrium through neuromuscular control. Coordination is a factor in balance, and for some activities agility is also important. Poor balance can lead to falls. Because balance decreases with age, it is important to maintain this component of physical fitness. In later years falls become a significant cause of morbidity and mortality. Regular activities such as t'ai chi can significantly improve and maintain balance.

BODY WEIGHT AND COMPOSITION

Body weight does not give an accurate measure of your body composition. A person with a high proportion of body fat may weigh less than one with a lean body mass. Muscle weighs more than fat and can indicate that you are overweight on a height and weight chart, whereas if your body composition has a high fat content you can appear to have an ideal weight but a less than optimal body composition. Your lean body mass is a better indication of your fitness level than body weight alone.

Health Benefits and Risks of Exercise

As previously discussed, regular exercise includes improvements in cardiorespiratory and musculoskeletal health. Improvement of your metabolism and psychological health can also occur with regular exercise, in addition to an increase in your longevity.[2] Exercise risks can be reduced by tailoring your exercise program specifically to your individual needs.

METABOLISM

Exercise along with diet can control obesity and reduce the insulin requirements of diabetics. A regular exercise program also helps to normalize blood triglycerides, increase high-density lipoproteins (good cholesterol) and lower low-density lipoproteins (bad cholesterol). The risk of osteoporosis can be reduced by endurance weight bearing that stresses the spine and femur, protecting the bone mineral density. Regular exercise aids in weight control and is a key part of any weight loss effort, changing your body fat into lean muscle.

PSYCHOLOGICAL STATE

A sense of well-being and a reduction in symptomatic depression and anxiety have been attributed to regular exercise. Exercise can also be used as a means of stress reduction that promotes relaxation. Moderate physical exercise can improve mental performance and improve mental fitness.

PHYSICAL EXERCISE AND LONGEVITY

Regular physical activity is associated with lower death rates for adults of any age.[1] It has been demonstrated that physical activity is effective in postponing mortality and enhancing longevity. A significantly lower death rate due to cardiovascular disease and cancer has been noted in those who exercise daily. It also appears that other causes of death are delayed with a higher level of physical fitness.

PREVENTION OF RISKS ASSOCIATED WITH EXERCISE

The risk of exercise-related musculoskeletal injuries can be minimized by adequate pre-exercise preparation and an appropriate exercise program. It is important that you have a comprehensive physical examination before beginning an exercise regimen. Your doctor of chiropractic can determine your current level of fitness and assist you to develop an individualized program with correct execution of exercises, adequate warm-up and cool-down periods, and an appropriate rate of exercise progression.

The Road toward Personal Fitness

It is important to address both mental and physical components of your personal fitness. We often attribute a separation of mind and body to Descartes, yet he stated that "the union of mind and body has to be acknowledged as being for us primary." Regular physical activity throughout life is important for maintaining a healthy body, enhancing psychological well-being, and preventing premature death.[1] Lifestyle strategies that promote fitness can help you change attitudes and activities of daily living in ways that promote your health and wellness. Your uniqueness as a human being lies in the conscious, deliberate, and creative aspects of your adaptation.[6] It is important that you have zestful work and play, frequently broken by complete mental and physical repose.

References

1. U.S. Department of Health and Human Services. *Healthy People 2010: Understanding and Improving Health*. 2nd ed. Washington, DC: U.S. Government Printing Office; November 2000.

2. Jamison JR. *Health Promotion for Chiropractic Practice*. Gaithersburg, MD: Aspen; 1991.

3. Rahe RH. Subjects' recent life changes and their near-future illness susceptibility. In: Lipowski ZJ, ed. *Advances in Pyschosomatic Medicine: Psychosocial Aspects of Physical Illness*. New York: S. Karger; 1973:2–40.

4. Jamison JR. *Maintaining Health in Primary Care: Guidelines for Wellness in the 21st Century*. St. Louis: Churchill Livingstone; 2001.

5. Gatterman MI. *Chiropractic Management of Spine Related Disorders*. 2nd ed. Baltimore: Lippincott Williams & Wilkins; 2004:364.

6. Dubos R. The credo of a biologist. In: Schwartz HS, ed. *Mental Health and Chiropractic*. New York: Sessions Publishers; 1973:286.

You Are What You Eat

Let food be your medicine.

Hippocrates

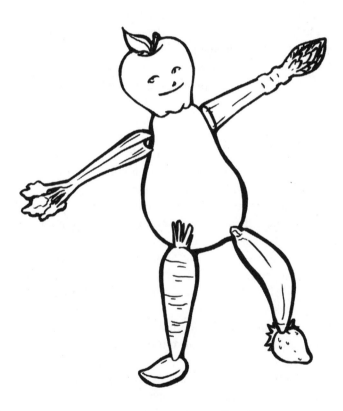

Nutrition is the relationship of foods to the health of the human body. Doctors of chiropractic have traditionally urged patients to pay attention to their diets in addition to exercising regularly.[1] Dietary deficiencies have been linked with various chronic diseases. A sound diet plays a major role in wellness and is promoted as part of your chiropractic wellness program.

Macronutrients

The macronutrients that make up your diet form the building blocks essential to the structure and function of your body. These macronutrients include water, carbohydrates, proteins, and fats.

Water is the medium in which other nutrients are found. Our bodies are approximately 60% water. Water is involved in almost every function in your body, including circulation, digestion, absorption, and elimination of waste. Water requirements are dependent on the climate in which you live, your activity level, and your diet. The average requirement is up to three quarts of water per day, including food and beverages. If you eat a diet high in fruits and vegetables, you will require less drinking water than if your diet is proportionately higher in meat and fats. Drinking water with meals dilutes your digestive juices; therefore, water is best consumed at several intervals during the day.

Carbohydrates are your main source of energy. Complex carbohydrates provide both an immediate and a slow release of energy since they are easily digested and consistently metabolized in the bloodstream. Refined carbohydrates and simple sugars should be avoided because they lack fiber, and their rapid release of energy is not sustained. They result in a spike in blood sugar followed by a sudden drop in response to insulin release. Refined carbohydrates and simple sugars are implicated in a variety of diseases, among them obesity, diabetes, cardiovascular problems, and tooth decay. If you consume higher levels of carbohydrates than immediately needed, the excess is converted to body fat.

Protein makes up about 20% of your body weight. It is a primary component of your muscles, hair, nails, skin, eyes, and internal organs—especially the heart muscle and brain. Protein is essential to your immune system, the hormones that regulate your metabolism, and your red blood cells that carry oxygen. A biochemical deficiency can occur when there is a lack of enzymes, the protein molecules that catalyze chemical reactions in your body. Excess consumption of protein, especially in the form of red meat, has been implicated in some forms of arthritis.

Fats are an important component of your diet, and at least a minimum intake is essential. Fat is primarily a form of energy reserve and provides insulation for your body. Your internal fatty tissues protect your vital organs from trauma and temperature change. Fats are an essential component of the cell membrane and are important in transporting other nutrients, such as the fat-soluble vitamins A, D, E, and K. Not all forms of fat offer equal health benefits. Unsaturated fats are preferable to saturated fats, and hydrogenated fats should especially be avoided. Essential fatty acids should be ingested in an appropriate ratio and are important for normal growth, healthy blood vessels and nerves, and to keep the skin and other tissues youthful and supple through their lubricating quality. Restricting dietary fat while maintaining adequate protein and complex carbohydrate intake is the best long-range approach to weight loss, maintenance of optimal body weight, and general good health for most individuals. Many problems are associated with excessive intake of dietary fat, including obesity, cardiovascular disease, and some forms of cancer.

MyPyramid

The U.S. government makes dietary recommendations in the form of a food pyramid in an endeavor to favorably modify your eating habits to reduce morbidity and mortality. The food pyramid, revised in 2005 by the U.S. Department of Agriculture (USDA), is only a broad guideline to healthy eating (Figure 5.1). Titled MyPyramid, this new food pyramid is designed to avoid a "one size fits all" solution to choosing a healthy diet. Completing an online survey gives you a broad guide to dietary recommendations based on your age, sex, and level of activity. MyPyramid is promoted as a "system of information to help consumers understand how to put nutrition into action." This interactive food guidance system replaces the old, flawed pyramid but doesn't convey enough information to help you make informed choices about your diet related to long-term health. Although designed to encourage good dietary habits that promote health and reduce the risk for major chronic diseases, the pyramid reflects the tense interplay of science and the powerful food industry. In addition to the USDA scientists and nutrition experts, intense lobbying from a variety of food industries helped shape the pyramid.

The food pyramid is a reflection of the nutrition advice assembled in the *Dietary Guidelines for Americans*, a document designed by the government to provide authoritative advice about good dietary habits that can "promote health and reduce risk for major chronic diseases." In *Dietary Guidelines for Americans*[2], recommendations for a healthy diet include the following:

- Emphasis on fruits, vegetables, whole grains, and fat-free or low-fat milk and milk products
- Inclusion of lean meats, poultry, fish, beans, eggs, and nuts
- Restriction of saturated fats, *trans* fats, cholesterol, salt (sodium), and added sugar

These dietary guidelines set standards for all federal nutrition programs, including school lunch programs. The guidelines influence how billions of dollars are spent each year, so even minor recommendations can hurt or help the food industry. Groups lobbying for representation on the panel that writes these guidelines include the National Dairy Council, United Fresh Fruit and Vegetable Association, Soft Drink Association, American Meat Institute, National Cattlemen's Beef Association, and Wheat Foods Council.

Figure 5.1 *MyPyramid*

Anatomy of MyPyramid

One size doesn't fit all

USDA's new MyPyramid symbolizes a personalized approach to healthy eating and physical activity. The symbol has been designed to be simple. It has been developed to remind consumers to make healthy food choices and to be active every day. The different parts of the symbol are described below.

Activity

Activity is represented by the steps and the person climbing them, as a reminder of the importance of daily physical activity.

Moderation

Moderation is represented by the narrowing of each food group from bottom to top. The wider base stands for foods with little or no solid fats or added sugars. These should be selected more often. The narrower top area stands for foods containing more added sugars and solid fats. The more active you are, the more of these foods can fit into your diet.

Personalization

Personalization is shown by the person on the steps, the slogan, and the URL. Find the kinds and amounts of food to eat each day at MyPyramid.gov.

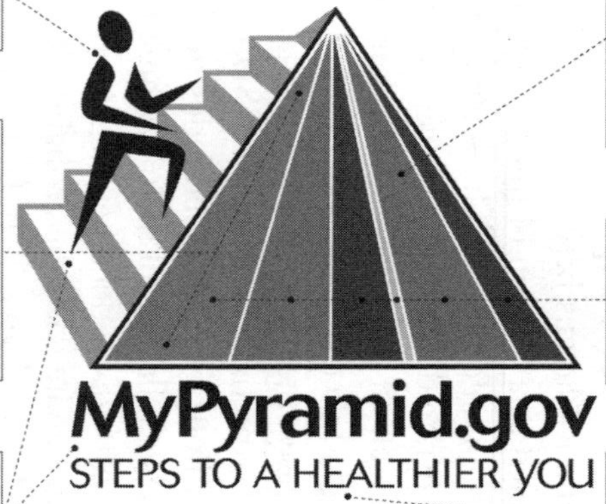

Proportionality

Proportionality is shown by the different widths of the food group bands. The widths suggest how much food a person should choose from each group. The widths are just a general guide, not exact proportions. Check the Web site for how much is right for you.

Variety

Variety is symbolized by the 6 color bands representing the 5 food groups of the Pyramid and oils. This illustrates that foods from all groups are needed each day for good health.

Gradual Improvement

Gradual improvement is encouraged by the slogan. It suggests that individuals can benefit from taking small steps to improve their diet and lifestyle each day.

MyPyramid.gov
STEPS TO A HEALTHIER YOU

GRAINS   VEGETABLES   FRUITS   OILS   MILK   MEAT & BEANS

USDA U.S. Department of Agriculture
Center for Nutrition Policy and Promotion
April 2005   CNPP-16

USDA is an equal opportunity provider and employer.

Courtesy of the U.S. Department of Agriculture, Center for Nutrition Policy and Promotion.

Micronutrients

Vitamin and Mineral Recommendations

Two groups of substances, vitamins and minerals, are classified as micronutrients. In addition to the food pyramid that makes recommendations for dietary macronutrients, guidelines for micronutrients are established by the Food and Nutrition Board (FNB) of the Institute of Medicine. The mandate of the FNB is to address issues of critical "importance pertaining to the safety and adequacy of the national food supply, to establish principles and guidelines for adequate nutrition, and to render authoritative judgment on the relationships among food intake, nutrition, and health."[3]

The original recommended daily allowances (RDAs) were purported to make recommendations for micronutrient requirements that were 50% greater than the average requirements for minerals and vitamins for a healthy person.[4] Through revision the RDAs have been replaced by Dietary Reference Intakes (DRIs). DRI values can be used for assessment, planning, education, and regulation. DRIs can be applied to assess the adequacy and wholesomeness of your individual dietary choices. This process provides information but is not conclusive for optimizing your nutritional requirements. If you seek vitality and wellness, amounts recommended for "average health" may not be sufficient for you. It is estimated that about 3% of people, even "healthy" ones, need more than the recommended amounts.[5] Healthcare practitioners, including doctors of chiropractic, have moved beyond a focused interest in the prevention of classical nutrient deficiencies. One set of values for specific nutrients needed for a given age, sex, and physiologic state may be unsatisfactory for meeting your individual needs.

The Reference Daily Intake is the value established by the Food and Drug Administration for use in nutrition labeling. Nutrition plays a fundamental role in promoting health and in avoiding and managing diet-related disease, so it is critical to your overall wellness. A higher value than the RDA, the optimal daily intake is designed to enhance general health and prevent disease. Since there are no government standards established for optimal requirements, your doctor of chiropractic must make decisions on the optimal amount for you as an individual, based on published studies and professional experience. These sources consider the following factors in determining your individual needs:

- Depletion of food nutrients through soil losses, chemicals, distance to market, processing, cooking, and storage
- Individual variability, such as stress, genetic requirements, environment, illness, drugs, age, and lifestyle
- Failure of government standards to adequately determine your needs

The Upper Limit value is the upper level of intake considered to be safe for use by adults and incorporates a safety factor. In some cases, greater values may be beneficial for the treatment of certain conditions and are not unsafe for specified lengths of time. It is important to remember that because of individual variability, recommended amounts may fall far short of what is necessary to promote your health and wellness.

Vitamins

Vitamins are organic substances present in varying quantities in specific foods. Each is absolutely necessary for your health and wellness. With few exceptions your body cannot synthesize vitamins, and they must be supplied in your diet or in dietary supplements. Some B vitamins can be made by your intestinal bacteria. It is important that if you have taken antibiotics that kill bacteria in the body, you replace the good bacteria in your gut. Vitamins have no caloric or energy value, but they are essential to your body as constituents of enzymes that function as catalysts in nearly all metabolic reactions. Each enzyme is specific to one biochemical reaction that would proceed very slowly, if at all, without them. Vitamins help to regulate metabolism, help to convert fat and carbohydrates into energy, and assist in forming bone and tissues. Vitamins are essential for growth, vitality, and health and are helpful in digestion, elimination, and resistance to disease. Depletion or deficiencies can lead to a variety of both specific nutritional disorders and general health problems, according to what vitamin is lacking in your diet.[5]

Vitamins are distinguished as being water-soluble or fat-soluble. The vitamin B complex and vitamin C are water-soluble. They are stable in raw foods but may be lost easily during cooking or processing. The water-soluble vitamins are not stored in the body to any degree, so they must be ingested regularly in your diet. Vitamins A, D, E, and K are fat-soluble. These fat-soluble vitamins can be stored in the body tissues, so you can function for longer periods of time without obtaining them from your diet. For this reason, however, toxic levels can occur more readily from excess intake of these vitamins.

Determining the recommended amounts of vitamins is an inexact science, and there is no way of predicting the exact requirements needed for optimal functioning of your body. Variables that affect nutritional requirements include climate, sex, age, state of health, body size, genetic makeup, and amount of activity. Where there is doubt that the requirements for certain nutrients are being met through the diet alone, supplements may be necessary to offset any deficiency. Recommended values for vitamins are presented in Table 5.1, but these values have nothing to do with maintaining vitality for a given individual. Needed amounts increase during even minor illnesses and during times of extra stress. Smoking and excess alcohol consumption increase the requirements for certain vitamins, as

Table 5.1 *Vitamin Recommendations*

Vitamin	1989 RDA	Current RDI[a]	New DRI[b]	Upper Limits[c]
Vitamin A	1000 RE	5000 IU	900 mcg (3000 IU)	3000 mcg (10,000 IU)
Vitamin C	60 mg	60 mg	90 mg	2000 mg
Vitamin D	10 mcg (400 IU)	400 IU	15 mcg (600 IU)	50 mcg (2000 IU)
Vitamin E	10 mg (15 IU)	30 IU (20 mg)	15 mg[d]	1000 mg
Vitamin K	80 mcg	80 mcg	120 mcg	ND
Thiamin	1.5 mg	1.5 mg	1.2 mg	ND
Riboflavin	1.8 mg	1.7 mg	1.3 mg	ND
Niacin	20 mg	20 mg	16 mg	35 mg
Vitamin B_6	2 mg	2 mg	1.7 mg	100 mg
Folate	200 mcg	400 mcg	400 mcg from food; 200 mcg synthetic[e]	1000 mcg (synthetic)
Vitamin B_{12}	2 mcg	6 mcg	2.4 mcg[f]	ND
Biotin	30–100 mcg	300 mcg	30 mcg	ND
Pantothenic acid	4–7 mg	10 mg	5 mg	ND
Choline	—	Not established	550 mg	3500 mg

[a]The Reference Daily Intake (RDI) is the value established by the Food and Drug Administration (FDA) for use in nutrition labeling. It was based initially on the highest 1968 recommended daily allowances (RDA) for each nutrient, to ensure that needs were met for all age groups.

[b]The Dietary Reference Intakes (DRI) are the most recent set of dietary recommendations established by the Food and Nutrition Board of the Institute of Medicine, 1997–2001. They replace previous RDAs and may be the basis for eventually updating the RDIs. The value shown here is the highest DRI for each nutrient.

[c]The Upper Limit (UL) is the upper level of intake considered to be safe for use by adults incorporating a safety factor. In some cases, lower ULs have been established for children.

[d]Historical vitamin E conversion factors were amended in the DRI report, so that 15 mg is defined as the equivalent of 22 IU of natural vitamin E or 33 IU of synthetic vitamin E.

[e]It is recommended that women of childbearing age obtain 400 mcg of synthetic folic acid from fortified breakfast cereals or dietary supplements, in addition to dietary folate.

[f]It is recommended that people over 50 meet the B_{12} recommendation through fortified foods or supplements, to improve bioavailability.

ND, Upper Limit not determined. No adverse effects were observed from high intakes of the nutrient.

Adapted from Council for Responsible Nutrition. Vitamin and mineral requirements. Available at http://www.crnusa.org/about_recs.html.

does excessive coffee and refined sugar intake. It should be remembered that recommended values for the average "healthy" person do not mean optimum amounts. Your wellness doctor of chiropractic can help you assess your specific vitamin requirements and make recommendations for diet and supplementation where necessary.

Minerals

Minerals are essential nutrients that exist in your body. Approximately 4% to 5% of your body weight is mineral matter, most of that in your skeleton. Minerals are vital to your overall mental and physical well-being. All tissues and internal fluids of living beings contain varying amounts of minerals. Minerals are constituents of your bones, teeth, soft tissues, muscles, blood, and nerve cells. They are present in enzymes and some vitamins. Minerals, although found in minute amounts in your body, are essential to your health. They are important factors in maintaining your physiological processes, strengthening your skeletal structures, and preserving the vigor of your heart and brain as well as your muscle and nerve systems.

Minerals act as catalysts for many biological reactions within your body, including muscle responses, the transmission of messages through your nervous system, digestion, and metabolism or utilization of nutrients in the foods you eat. Minerals are also essential in the production of hormones. All the minerals needed by your body must be supplied by the food you eat or through nutritional supplements. Recommended amounts of required minerals are presented in Table 5.2.

Like vitamins, minerals contain no calories or energy in themselves but are necessary to assist the body in energy production. Although your body can manufacture some vitamins, it cannot make minerals. The minerals that we need come from the earth, and if a mineral nutrient is not contained in the soil, it will not be in the food grown in that soil. Loss of topsoil, continual replanting without enriching the soil, or the use of fertilizers that contain only nitrogen, phosphorus, and potassium (all of which stimulate plant growth) and not other important minerals mean that your food may not contain all the minerals necessary for your health. Fruits and vegetables grown in rich, well-nourished soil have the essential minerals we need for our health and wellness. Refinement and processing of foods further decrease the mineral content of your food. The molasses left after refining sugar, for example, which is rich in minerals, is usually fed to animals. Refined sugar lacks the cofactors necessary to metabolize the sugar. The same is true for the milling of wheat, refining of corn, and polishing of rice. Obtaining the full spectrum of essential minerals is further compromised when absorption is less than optimal. With digestive difficulties, trace minerals such as chromium and zinc may be poorly absorbed and deficiency symptoms may develop quite rapidly.

Table 5.2 *Mineral Requirements*

Mineral	RDA 1989	DRI 1997-98
Zinc	12 mg (females); 15 mg (males)	—
Copper	1.5–3 mg	—
Chromium	50–200 mcg	—
Selenium	55 mcg (females); 70 mcg males	—
Iodine	150 mcg	—
Molybdenum	75–250 mcg	—
Manganese	2–5 mg	—
Magnesium	280 mg (females); 350 mg (males)	310–320 mg (females) 400–420 mg (males) 360–400 mg (pregnant) 310–360 mg (lactating)
Calcium	800 mg	1000–1200 mg 1000–1300 mg (pregnant, lactating)
Iron	15 mg (females); 10 mg (males)	—
Phosphorus	800 mg 1200 mg (11–24 yrs, pregnancy, and lactating)	700 mg 1000–1300 mg (pregnant and lactating)
Potassium	3500 mg	—
Sodium	2240 mg	—

Adapted from Seaman DR. *Clinical Nutrition for Pain, Inflammation, and Tissue Healing*. Hendersonville, NC: NutrAnalysis; 1998.

Most minerals are not destroyed by heat, but some are soluble in water and therefore are leached out during the cooking process.

Special electrolyte minerals, including sodium, potassium, and chloride, help regulate the fluid and acid-base balance of your body. Other minerals are an essential part of enzymes that catalyze biochemical reactions and aid the production of energy or participate in metabolism. Some minerals assist in nerve transmission, muscle contraction, cell permeability, and blood and tissue formation.

Some toxic metals can cause harm when found in relatively high concentrations in your body. These are primarily lead, mercury, aluminum, and cadmium. These heavy metals are found in the atmosphere, rivers, food sources, and many industrial products. Metal poisoning primarily affects the metabolic enzymes, brain, and nervous system, but other body functions can be affected as well. Health problems can occur when high amounts are present from either excessive intake of minerals or a reduced ability to eliminate them.

Many minor and major problems can arise from mineral deficiencies. Osteoporosis is the best known, a deficiency of bone minerals due to low calcium intake, lack of vitamin D, and insufficient protein that forms the matrix for laying down the calcium. Low calcium, potassium, and magnesium levels and high sodium intake contribute to hypertension. Magnesium deficiency is associated with muscle spasms and nerve-related pain and heart disease. Low zinc and selenium levels compromise the immune system, making you prone to infection. Subtle mineral deficiencies are difficult to diagnose. Analysis of the hair shaft (hair analysis) gives an indication of the long-term status of minerals in the body, but remains controversial. Accepted as a means of detecting heavy metal content, it has not been readily accepted as a means of indicating health status or specific mineral deficiencies. Your wellness chiropractor can advise you on this procedure.

The healthiest approach to ensuring optimum levels of micronutrients in your body is to get the majority of them from wholesome foods. Eating a variety of foods, with a lot of organic, local produce and whole grains, is a good start. Avoiding refined and processed foods that have poor mineral and vitamin content is helpful. Eliminating foods containing refined sugar, excess caffeine, and alcohol, all of which increase the requirement for micronutrients, is a major step in improving your nutritional status. Orienting yourself to a healthy diet by eating a variety of wholesome foods will assure you the basics of good nutrition.

Developing Healthy Eating Habits

Developing healthy eating habits may be just as important as what you eat. A relaxed atmosphere promotes digestion, as does eating slowly. Habits to avoid include overeating, undereating, eating late in the evening, and restricting the variety of your food.

Overeating

Overeating is one of the most common and dangerous eating habits. Often we overeat, seeking the nutrients necessary to metabolize the food we ingest. When empty calories are consumed, there is a craving for more food to provide the necessary missing micronutrients. In this sense overeating is a malnutrition disorder. Celebrations, holidays, and parties too often stress eating to excess. Overeating is often influenced by parents and family members, with a great many emotional and psychological factors starting in the early years. Obesity is a contributing factor in many other diseases. The overconsumption of food causes stress to the digestive tract and other organs. Moderation in eating, along with emphasis on healthy food, is a very important habit to develop.

Undereating

Undereating is a serious health problem, especially in the young adolescent. Anorexia nervosa and bulimia are serious disorders related to undereating that can be life threatening. *Anorexia* literally means "loss of appetite," and anorexia nervosa means not eating because of "nervous" or psychological problems. Bulimia is voluntary vomiting so as not to absorb calories and add weight. Undereating usually has a strong stress or psychological component. All forms of undereating, skipping meals, or eating only limited foods can lead to poor nutrition and eventually to deficiencies of calories, protein, essential fats, vitamins, and minerals. Symptoms of undereating include lack of energy and subsequent weakness, malnourishment of internal organs, skin and nail problems, and hair loss. People who undereat are often overly concerned about obesity and their body image. The consumption of adequate calories to promote wellness is a healthy habit.

Eating Late

Eating just before bedtime may be a common problem if you consume too few calories during the day, or if your daily schedule is so busy that eating is put off until later. Eating just before going to bed is not helpful to digestion and is not necessarily beneficial to sleep. Food eaten late at night may just sit in the stomach, undigested through the night, so that you wake up full and sluggish. Eating earlier in the day is a habit that promotes vitality and a sense of well-being.

Restricting Your Variety of Food

Restricting your variety of food creates a diet that is more prone to deficiencies. This inflexibility is often based on a preference for certain tastes. Teenagers and elderly people are more likely to indulge in this habit. Different cultures have different tastes, and a lack of adventure or fear can create an attitude that does not allow you to be open to new foods. A diet limited to fast food such as hamburgers, hot dogs, French fries, and sodas (common to adolescents) or tea and toast (in the older age group) does not promote healthy nutrition. A diet limited to meat and potatoes lacks the freshness and vitality found in natural foods. Ideally, you should eat a variety of foods, and a healthy plan is to introduce new foods when the opportunity arises.

Environmental Aspects of Nutrition

The deteriorating environment compromises your health through pollution of your body from pesticide residuals and industrial chemicals, food additives, and genetically modified (GM) foods. We have also discussed overuse of artificial fertilizers that do not adequately replace micronutrients in chronically depleted soil.

Although chemicals can have a beneficial role in our current consumer-oriented society, corporations that manufacture chemicals and the food industry benefit more than consumers do. Cheaper food at the expense of health and wellness is false economy. Everyone needs to be aware of and concerned about the impact of industrial chemicals on our health. Constant exposure to even small amounts of toxic materials is not risk free. Chemicals are tested for their effect on small laboratory animals whose short life spans do not allow for the study of the effects of the chemicals' accumulation over time. Accumulation occurs when chemicals don't break down. Their presence in the body can cause repeated insults, leading to chronic diseases. You don't produce all of the enzymes necessary to break down the multitude of synthetic chemicals bombarding your body, nor can you metabolize and excrete them. The carcinogenicity of many chemicals is well documented, and not all cancer-causing chemicals have been subjected to research studies. Many pesticides, fungicides, herbicides, and preservative chemicals can cause liver disease as well as cancer. Though not immediately life threatening, chemical exposure can lead to allergies and chemical sensitivities that cause much suffering and distress.

The chemical industry and agribusinesses work together to promote the use of chemical fertilizers and pesticides. It has become increasingly more difficult to obtain food that doesn't contain harmful chemical residuals. The herbicide Roundup, for example, has been spliced into soybean plants. Most soybeans in the United States have been GM in this manner. If you are a label reader, you will know how difficult it is to avoid products containing soy. When you have no other option but to buy conventionally grown produce, it is important to make sure you wash off any external residual pesticides.

Whereas contaminants such as pesticides and fertilizers accidentally get into food as residues, additives are deliberately introduced to food, both during processing and as ingredients, to improve flavor, color, or shelf life. The food industry uses approximately 3,000 different food additives in various packaged and preserved foods. These include emulsifiers, buffers, and natural and artificial flavoring and coloring. Non-nutritional reasons for the inclusion of additives in processed foods include the following:

- To prolong shelf life
- To make food more convenient

- To improve flavor
- To improve consumer acceptance

The use of hormones to fatten cattle or to induce them to produce more milk is also controversial, as is the addition of antibiotics to animal feed. Although these practices are of benefit to the food industry, there is little justification for their use on the basis of consumer health. Addition of antibiotics to animal feed can leave residuals that may cause a reaction if you are allergic to penicillin or are sulfa sensitive.

Packaging can also contribute to food contamination. The use of plastic wrap to package food can leave dangerous polyvinyl chloride (PVC) residuals in food when the wrap is heated to seal the package. The use of heat releases PVC as a gas. This threatens the consumer with free radical formation, cellular irritation, increased allergies, and the potential for the genesis of cancer cells.

Genetically Modified Food

The application of biotechnology to modify food has caused concern related to health. Not all biotechnology is harmful, and in general terms it has been used for centuries, in the sense of using organisms or their components, such as enzymes, to make products such as wine, cheese, beer, and yogurt. GM foods, on the other hand, combine genes from different organisms into what is known as recombinant DNA. The resulting organism is said to be *genetically modified, genetically engineered*, or *transgenic*. GM products include animal feed, foods, and food ingredients. The most common transgenic crops that have been GM with herbicides and insecticides are soybeans, corn, cotton, and canola. Other GM crops grown commercially are sweet potatoes and rice.

Controversies that surround GM food include the following:[6]

- *Safety:* Potential human health issues include the introduction of allergens into previously safe food and the transfer of antibiotic resistance markers. GM foods that can cause food allergies include tomatoes modified with fish genes. Environmental issues are the unintended transfer of transgenes through cross-pollination, unknown effects on other organisms (e.g., soil microbes), and loss of flora and fauna biodiversity.
- *Ethics:* Unless GM foods are carefully labeled, you can consume animal genes in plants and vice versa.
- *Labeling:* Labeling is not mandatory in some countries, including the United States. The mixing of GM crops with non-GM crops confounds labeling attempts.

- *Societal:* New advances may be skewed to the interest of developed countries, with domination of world food production by a few companies. This can lead to dependence on industrialized nations by developing countries, with foreign exploitation of natural resources.

GM foods continue to remain controversial. Current foods that have been altered genetically include soybeans, corn, tomatoes, potatoes, sugar beets, farm-raised salmon, wheat, rice, and canola. When such foods are not appropriately labeled, it is not possible to know when to avoid substances that may cause an allergic reaction. The safest course of action is to eat foods labeled as not GM.

Irradiation of Foods

Irradiation of foods means that they have been exposed to penetrating radiation. Irradiation damages the natural enzymes in foods. Irradiation of fats creates free radicals, causing the fats to become rancid. Free radicals have been implicated in many cancers. Studies of irradiated foods have shown that irradiation can cause damage to the kidneys and liver. Irradiated foods at some processing plants include meats, fruits, vegetables, and juices.

Organic Foods

Understanding the difference between natural and organic foods is important. Natural foods are not synthetically produced. Although they are not modified, they may be highly processed with harmful chemicals, such as those used in refining sugar. The requirements for organic status vary from state to state. California has the most stringent requirements for organic certification. In most jurisdictions, *organic* means grown without

- Pesticides or fertilizers
- Transgenic ingredients (GM organisms)
- Irradiation in the processing
- Fertilizer from human sewage/sludge

The safest way to avoid unwanted contaminants in your diet is to seek out organic sources of food. More local supermarkets are carrying organic foods, and you can request that they do so if they currently do not. You can also demand that their growers and distributors label foods that have been GM. Many local farm stands and markets specialize in fresh seasonal organic produce. Purchasing your foods from markets that specialize in organic foods is possible, and by shopping around you can find the least expensive sources. Growing your own fruits and vegetables can ensure that they are safe and wholesome if you are in an area where this is feasible. Even a patio garden can be helpful—just requiring sun, water, organic soil, and a little determination.

Important foods to eat organic are as follows:

- Baby food (the young are susceptible to pesticides)
- Cherries
- Celery
- Apricots and grapes
- Soybeans
- Potatoes
- Raisins
- Strawberries
- Rice
- Milk
- Bananas
- Green beans
- Peaches
- Apples
- Cucumbers
- Meat, fish, and poultry

Food Additives to Avoid

Although many food additives are safe, some should be carefully avoided. These include the following:

- *Acesulfame:* An artificial sweetener found in sugar-free baked goods, gelatin desserts, soft drinks, and chewing gum.
- *Artificial colorings:* Usually found in foods of low nutritional value, such as candy, soda pop, gelatin desserts, and so forth.
- *Aspartame:* Artificial sweetener (Equal, NutriSweet) found in diet foods. Aspartame has been linked to some cancers.
- *Cyclamate:* An artificial sweetener banned in 1970. Thought to increase the potency of other carcinogens and to harm the testes.
- *Olestra:* A fat substitute that is not absorbed by the body but runs through it. Olestra can cause diarrhea, loose stools, abdominal cramps, flatulence,

and other adverse effects. It reduces the body's ability to absorb fat-soluble nutrients that reportedly reduce the risk of cancer and heart disease.

- *Potassium bromate:* Increases the volume and texture of bread. Bromate causes cancer in animals. Bromate has been banned worldwide except in Japan and the United States. It is rarely used in California because a cancer warning might be required on the label.
- *Propyl gallate:* An antioxidant that retards spoilage of fats and oils. Used in vegetable oil, meat products, potato sticks, chicken soup base, and chewing gum.
- *Saccharin:* An artificial sweetener found in diet products, soft drinks (especially fountain drinks at restaurants), and in sugar substitute packets (Sweet'N Low). Saccharin has been linked to cancer of the urinary bladder.
- *Sodium nitrite:* A preservative, flavoring, and coloring agent used in bacon, ham, frankfurters, luncheon meats, smoked fish, and corned beef. Adding nitrite to food can lead to the formation of small amounts of potent cancer-causing chemicals (nitrosamines), particularly in fried bacon.
- *Stevia:* A natural, high-potency sweetener used as a sugar substitute. Stevia has not been approved as a food additive in Canada and the United States because it may be converted to steviol, a mutagenic compound that may promote cancer. Small amounts of stevia may be safe, but it is inappropriate to endorse wide use of this sweetener.

Maintaining Health and Promoting Wellness Through Nutrition

The *nut* in *nutrition* does not mean you are a health nut in attempting to promote health and wellness by eating a healthy diet. What can seem a formidable task can become second nature when you seek to change eating habits over time. As with modifying any unhealthy behavior, it is important to not make too many dramatic changes all at once. With the multitude of ways you can change your diet for the better, a slow to moderate pace in making changes is recommended. If you wish to eat healthier, you need to change what and how you eat as a habit rather than approaching it as going on a diet.[5]

A number of ways to make your diet healthier are outlined in Table 5.3. Perhaps the most significant is to read labels carefully. If you can't identify an ingredient or pronounce it, you need to find out what it is. Consuming moderate amounts of all foods while gradually eliminating those that are unhealthy is the most prudent way to begin. Avoiding foods that you have consumed for a long

Table 5.3 *Making Your Diet Healthier*

Read labels.

Consume moderate amounts of fat (including essential fatty acids) and red meat.

Consume less fried foods. (Bake, broil, or boil instead.)

Avoid all hydrogenated oils. (This type of fat is not used by the body and increases the risk of cardiovascular disease.)

Avoid refined sugar. (Look for hidden sugar in prepared foods.)

Avoid excess coffee and alcohol. (Both add stress to your system and require additional micronutrients for their metabolism.)

Consume recommended amounts of raw fruit and vegetables. (Substitute these foods to avoid excess fat, protein, and simple sugars.)

Eat whole-grain cereals (brown rice, whole wheat, oats, barley, etc.).

Replace red meats with fish and poultry. (Some fish contain healthy oils.)

Seek protein from nuts, seeds, and beans. (Eating these foods helps you reduce unhealthy fat while maintaining adequate protein.)

Drink adequate amounts of water. (Water is the medium in which all other nutrients are found.)

Include whole foods that contain fiber. (This prevents constipation and gastrointestinal disease.)

Ensure that you are ingesting sufficient micronutrients to promote health and wellness. (Supplements may be required.)

Consume appropriate amount of calories for your body weight. (Obesity is a health hazard contributing to many diseases.)

Adapted from Haas EM. *Staying Healthy with Nutrition*. Berkeley, CA: Celestial Arts; 1992.

period may be best approached by decreasing their amounts rather than eliminating these foods altogether. Hydrogenated oils, refined sugar, coffee, and alcohol can all be reduced with the object of avoiding some or all of these altogether. Substituting recommended amounts of raw fruits and vegetables for excess amounts of fat, protein, and simple sugars is a reasonable goal. Eating more whole-grain cereals (brown rice, whole wheat, oats, and barley) is healthier than eating highly refined and processed foods. Replacing red meats with fish and poultry and eating nuts, seeds, and beans provides adequate protein while helping to reduce unhealthy fat.

Ensuring a sufficient quantity of water and fiber is as important to health and wellness as adequate intake of nutrients. Above all, it is essential to ingest sufficient micronutrients so that you are satiated by the appropriate amount of calories for your body weight. Ideally, dietary recommendations should be achieved through informed food choices, but nutrient supplements may be necessary when individual deficiencies are identified. Guidance for staying healthy through nutrition can be provided by your doctor of chiropractic.

References

1. Seaman DR. *Clinical Nutrition for Pain, Inflammation, and Tissue Healing*. Hendersonville, NC: NutrAnalysis; 1998.

2. Department of Health and Human Services (HHS) and the Department of Agriculture (USDA). *Dietary Guidelines for Americans 2005*. Available at: http://www.health.gov/dietaryguidelines/dga2005/document.

3. Institute of Medicine. Food and Nutrition Board. Available at: http://www.iom.edu/CMS/3788.aspx.

4. Jamison JR. *Health Promotion for Chiropractic Practice*. Gaithersburg, MD: Aspen; 1991:29.

5. Haas EM. *Staying Healthy with Nutrition*. Berkeley, CA: Celestial Arts; 1992.

6. U.S. Department of Energy Office of Science, Office of Biological and Environmental Research. Genetically modified foods and organisms. Available at: http://www.ornl.gov/sci/techresources/HumanGenome/elsi/gmfood.shtml.

Chapter 6

Spinal Health Promotion

Ron Kirk

The spine is the organ of posture, the lifeline of the body.

Fred Illi

C hances are, if you are like most people, when you think about chiropractic, the first thing that comes to mind is your spinal health, and for good reason. Spinal health promotion is indeed one of the key areas of focus for doctors of chiropractic. Every year millions of individuals participate in spinal health promotion partnering relationships with doctors of chiropractic. When you seek chiropractic services, your doctor of chiropractic will help you improve the level of your spinal health, utilizing a balanced, multifaceted approach. Initially he or she will make a comprehensive assessment of your spinal health status and, when necessary, adjust localized areas of spinal misalignment and joint restriction called spinal subluxations. Your doctor of chiropractic will then work with you to develop an active, personalized program of spinal exercises and ergonomic and lifestyle recommendations designed to help you improve your spinal health and prevent injury and disability. Often doctors of chiropractic will also assist you in developing nutritional and stress management plans aimed at optimizing your spinal health and overall wellness.

First let's discuss some of the assessments your doctor of chiropractic will perform to help you determine the status of your spinal health. If you have a specific spinal complaint, these assessments will usually begin with a history aimed at identifying your problem and the behaviors or lifestyle risk factors that may affect your spinal health negatively or positively. Your doctor will ask you about particular problem areas where your back, head, and neck may feel painful or uncomfortable. He or she will begin by asking you standardized questions about the nature of your spinal complaint: when it began, what makes it better or worse, how often it occurs, its nature or quality, how severe or painful it is on a scale of one to ten, and so on.

In searching for causes of your problem, your doctor will usually question you regarding your type of work and ergonomic environment. He or she will focus on spinal health risk factors such as frequent participation in heavy lifting or prolonged periods of sitting while word processing. Doctors of chiropractic often ask probing questions regarding posture in order to discern whether you have developed the prevalent and very detrimental habit of slouching. In addition to your standing or sitting postural habits, your chiropractor will want to know about your sleeping postures and the type of mattress or bed you are currently using. Commonly your doctor will also question you regarding the quality of your work environment, including the existence of mechanical or toxic hazards in your work area. The quality of our work and home environment and our habitual patterns of behavior have a major impact on the quality of our spinal health.

In taking your history, your doctor may also ask questions regarding your levels of stress at home or at work. Unresolved stress strongly influences our spinal columns, often producing paraspinal muscle tension and spinal joint restriction or locking. Because doctors of chiropractic approach health promotion comprehensively, they usually will also question you about your eating habits, including specific foods and nutrients, which affect your spinal health. Commonly your doctor will also question you regarding the use of tobacco and excessive amounts of alcohol. Substance abuse has detrimental effects on your spinal health as well as your overall wellness.

After conducting a thorough history, your chiropractor will usually begin a chiropractic physical examination in order to further assess the health of your spinal column. He or she will palpate your spine for areas of spinal tenderness, muscle spasm, joint restriction, and misalignment. These restricted and often tender areas are what doctors of chiropractic call *spinal subluxations*. They may also be known as *articular dysfunction* or *spinal motion segment dysfunction*. Doctors of chiropractic have extensive training in locating and correcting spinal dysfunction. Subluxations are of particular concern to your doctor, because these structural and functional lesions can interfere with harmonious functioning of your nervous system, thus producing far-reaching effects on your health.

In addition to palpating your spinal column for the presence of spinal dysfunction and spinal distortions such as scoliosis, your doctor may assess your posture utilizing various types of plumb-line devices or photographic computerized systems. Postural assessment is vital to you and your chiropractor because the spinal column is the central balancing and postural structure of your body. Poor posture often leads to compromised spinal function, spinal subluxations, and other posture-related disorders. Because the spine is the central support structure for many of our organs, poor posture can also compromise important visceral functions such as breathing and digestion. Your doctor of chiropractic will help you assess your posture in order to make improvements in this vital component of spinal and overall health. To maintain your balance in the standing position with a minimum of energy, the joints of your spine and lower extremities must be aligned. A gravity line using a plumb line is often utilized to determine deviations from ideally aligned posture. Figure 6.1 illustrates the points of your body through which an ideal gravity line should fall.

Additionally, your doctor will often screen for spinal pathologies or structural assymetries through the use of x-rays. Most doctors of chiropractic will take x-rays of your spine to check for the presence of spinal subluxations, scolioses, structural assymetries, and pathologies that may compromise spinal structure and function and complicate care. In many instances it is important for your doctor to rule out spinal pathologies such as fractures or malignancies before delivering adjustments to your spinal column.

Many doctors of chiropractic will use a variety of other tests to check for spinal subluxations, including checks for leg length imbalance and muscle weakness. Doctors of chiropractic often utilize instruments to assess spinal muscle tone imbalances or skin temperature variation in areas adjacent to your spinal column. Additionally it is very common for doctors of chiropractic to use orthopedic tests to assess your spinal column for its structural and functional integrity and the presence of nerve root lesions. Neurological tests are often employed because the cranium and spinal column house and protect the central nervous system, and disorders of these protective encasements can affect neurological functions.

After your doctor of chiropractic has made comprehensive assessments of your spinal health, he or she will develop a plan for your care, which may include corrective phases to address initial problems and stabilize your spinal health and a wellness phase of care aimed at optimizing your spinal health. These phases of care are usually part of a continuum or progression of care and merge into one another.

Early in corrective care, your doctor will usually focus on a series of adjustments to your spinal column aimed at correcting spinal misalignments and loosening restricted areas of spinal subluxation. Usually as these areas of spinal dysfunction become better aligned and more freely movable, the frequency of adjustments will decrease to a level at which you will get your spinal alignment and balance checked from time to time and adjusted when necessary to maintain optimal function. Doctors of chiropractic are highly skilled in administering adjustments to the spinal column. The adjustments free restricted or immobilized joints that can degenerate progressively through a process called *immobilization degeneration*.[1] Joints are designed for motion; when immobilized, they often become inflamed, and joint capsules become constricted. Spinal adjustments realign spinal joints, stretch constricted muscles and ligaments, and bring fresh circulation to the area. This helps to remove inflammatory debris from the restricted joint. Furthermore, adjustments also produce very strong motion feedback stimulus into the

Figure 6.1 *The points of your body through which an ideal gravity line should fall.*

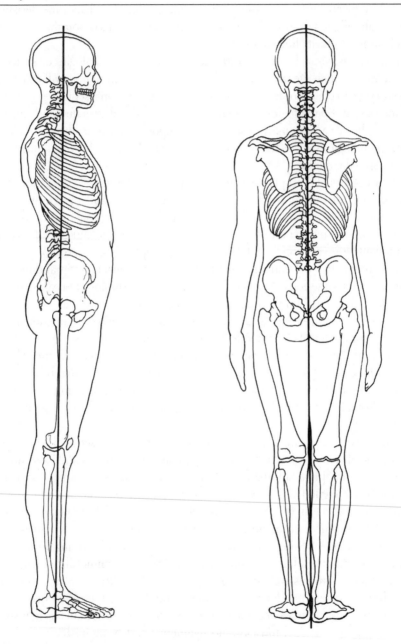

Reprinted with permission from Gatterman MI. *Chiropractic Management of Spine Related Disorders*. 2nd ed. Baltimore: Lippincott Williams & Wilkins; 2004.

Figure 6.2 *A chiropractic adjustment with the patient lying on her side.*

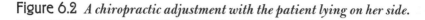

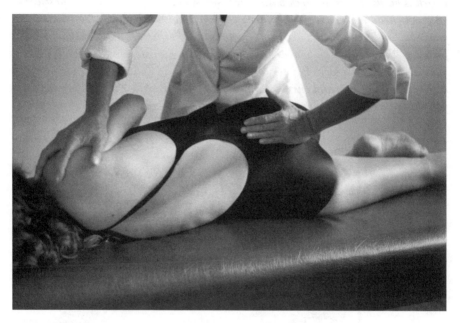

Reprinted with permission from Gatterman MI. *Chiropractic Management of Spine Related Disorders*. 2nd ed. Baltimore: Lippincott Williams & Wilkins; 2004.

nervous system and reduce the firing of patterns of chronic pain feedback. Figure 6.2 illustrates a chiropractic adjustment with the patient lying on her side.

Simultaneous with the series of spinal adjustments, your doctor will make you aware of specific exercises that can help you to correct postural distortions and structural misalignments that you may have. It is extremely important that you become active in your spinal health promotion plan in the same way that you are empowered to take responsibility for your dental health and overall health and fitness by regularly engaging in excellent health promotion habits. Because slouched, stooped posture is becoming more pronounced in our increasingly sedentary society, your performance of daily postural exercises is vital to your spinal health (see Appendix A).

Your doctor will demonstrate some simple exercises, such as the Posture Pod from the Straighten Up program. When practiced regularly, these and similar exercises will help you to improve your posture and strengthen core stabilizing muscles surrounding your spine, abdomen, hips, and pelvic areas. These exercises are aimed at reducing your tendency to stoop or slouch, an unhealthy habit. Slouching produces excessive strain in your upper back and neck muscles. In slouched

Figure 6.3 *In A, the ideal gravity line falls through the center of the head, which is balanced on the neck with a minimum of energy. In slouched posture (B), your head moves excessively forward, your shoulders drop forward, and your chest collapses downward, making breathing difficult. As your head moves forward, the gravity line moves backward, causing tension in the muscles of your neck that must work harder to balance your head on your neck. This shift also increases the normal curves of your spine, compressing the vital organs of your body and affecting your overall health and well-being.*

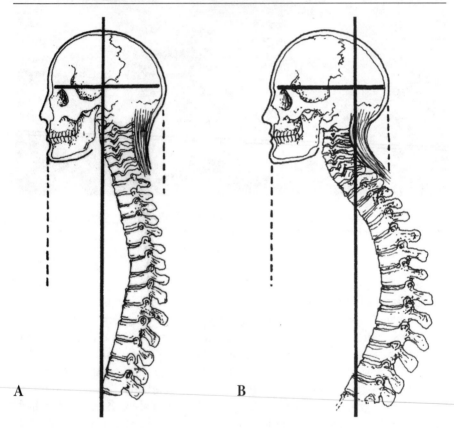

A   B

Reprinted with permission from Gatterman MI. *Chiropractic Management of Spine Related Disorders*. 2nd ed. Baltimore: Lippincott Williams & Wilkins; 2004.

posture, your head moves excessively forward, your shoulders drop forward, and your chest collapses downward, making breathing difficult (Figure 6.3). If this postural pattern is not corrected, it often leads to increasing spinal disability with advancing age. People who slouch are prone to headaches and a host of neck, shoulder, and upper limb disorders.[2]

Your doctor will often recommend specific exercises, including shoulder and head retraction exercises, to assist you in improving slouched posture. Additionally, he or she may prescribe specific stretching and strengthening exercises for correction or reduction of other patterns of spinal distortion. Many doctors of chiropractic have rehabilitation suites or centers in their offices with specialized exercise equipment designed to help you improve your spinal health. Additionally, your doctor of chiropractic will encourage you to engage in an active lifestyle with plenty of exercise to help prevent osteoporosis and maintain high levels of physical fitness. Ultimately, the responsibility for actively promoting your spinal health rests upon your shoulders as you work in partnership with your doctor of chiropractic. Active, physically fit people experience improved spinal health and overall wellness and receive the extra benefits of increased physical vitality and improved mental health (see Chapter 4).[3]

In addition to performance of spinal exercises for postural improvement, your doctor may recommend alterations to your ergonomic environment to help you improve your spinal health. Ergonomics is the study of the fit between us and our workplace. Chiropractors are trained in sound ergonomic principles, practices, and evaluation (see Chapter 7). Your doctor of chiropractic may suggest strategies for improving your work environment, such as improving the type of chair you sit in, the eye level of your computer monitor, or the level of your wrist and hands while working at your computer keyboard. He or she may also recommend particular exercises for highly important ergonomic breaks and offer suggestions or devices and supports for optimizing your postural balance when you work.

While at work or in our homes, many of us experience significant levels of another extremely important health factor—stress. Deadlines, divergent perspectives, and differences of opinion and personality can build conflict and cause unresolved distress. If you are having difficulty managing stress at work or in other areas of your life, your doctor may recommend some simple stress management strategies for you, such as increasing your level of physical activity or finding higher levels of emotional support. If the problems you are dealing with are more complex, he or she may also be able to assist you by referring you to a professional specializing in stress management or psychological counseling. As mentioned earlier, unresolved stress affects spinal health detrimentally due in part to increased muscle tension around the spinal column and restriction of spinal mobility. Often patients receiving spinal adjustments report a sense of release from stress and associated tension in areas around the spinal column.

In summary, doctors of chiropractic are highly skilled at assisting people in increasing their levels of spinal health. Your doctor of chiropractic will conduct a very thorough assessment of your spinal health, including a health history, a thorough chiropractic examination, and a postural and muscle balance evaluation. He or she will search for and correct areas of restricted motion and misalignment in your spinal column called spinal subluxations. After you receive chiropractic adjustments, your spinal column should move more freely and comfortably. Additionally, your doctor of chiropractic will encourage you to become actively involved in spinal health promotion by teaching you specific exercises for postural improvement and core stability. He or she will offer exercise, nutritional, ergonomic, and stress management advice as a mentor where appropriate.

Ideally, you and your doctor of chiropractic will form a health promotion partnership. In this partnership you will play the most prominent role by gaining knowledge of health promotion practices, engaging actively in a healthy lifestyle, and taking responsibility for promoting your spinal and overall wellness. Increasingly, studies indicate that individuals who consistently partner with their doctors of chiropractic in positive health promotion habits and systematic chiropractic care enjoy a higher quality of life and decreased healthcare costs and hospitalizations.[4,5]

References

1. Liebenson C. Pathogenesis of chronic back pain. *J Manipulative Physiol Ther*. 1992;15:303.

2. Szeto GPY, Straker L, Raine S. A field comparison of neck and shoulder postures in symptomatic and asymptomatic office workers. *Appl Ergon*. 2002;33:75–84.

3. Blair SN, et al. *Active Living Every Day*. Champaign, IL: Human Kinetics; 2001.

4. Rupert RL, Manello D, Sandefur R. Maintenance care: health promotion services administered to U.S. chiropractic patients aged 65 and older, part II. *J Manipulative Physiol Ther*. 2000;25(1):10–19.

5. Rupert RL. A survey of practice patterns and the health promotion and prevention attitudes of U.S. chiropractors. Maintenance care: part I. *J Manipulative Physiol Ther*. 2000;25(1):1–9.

Chapter 7

Performance Enhancement

The human body is a multilinked mechanical system that adapts to the complexity of motor functioning and kinetic demands.

Meridel I. Gatterman

Optimal performance utilizes techniques that are more effective and less demanding of energy.[1] Performance enhancement comes from application of the scientific principles of kinesiology. *Kinesiology* is the discipline that studies movement. The term is derived from the Greek word *kine*, meaning movement or motion. Kinesiology that analyzes human movement should not be confused with *Applied Kinesiology*, which is a chiropractic technique system that uses muscle testing to diagnose various conditions. When we think of performance enhancement, we often limit it to improving athletic or military performance. It is equally important that movements in everyday living be evaluated for efficiency. Becoming more proficient and skillful at activities of daily living contributes significantly to your health and wellness.

The Science of Human Movement

The human mechanism must meet both the static and dynamic demands of extremely diversified activities. These range all the way from sitting and standing to specialized skills used in work and recreational activities. The physical laws governing human mechanics are universal. To help you improve performance, the mechanisms of physics can be applied to analyze both your work and recreational activities. The discipline of biomechanics is a subset of kinesiology that studies the human body to make necessary physical adaptations. Approaching the human body as a machine does not, however, present the whole picture. Understanding the physiology and psychology of movement is also necessary when applying the science of kinesiology to your overall performance. Factors that should be considered in the application of kinesiological principles to your activities include the following:

- The facts and principles of the basic sciences that contribute to the science of kinesiology
- Your specific activities
- Problems related to gravity, stress and strain on body parts, and muscular strength and tonus in the determination of optimal postures
- Your individual skills
- Psychological considerations that can improve your performance
- Irregular and unusual performance related to your individual body

Changing Your Environment Can Affect Your Performance

The physical and social environment in which you live contributes significantly to your lifestyle, and affects your work and play. Your performance both in the workplace and during recreational activities can be improved by modifying your environment in addition to improving your physical skill. Your doctor of chiropractic can make recommendations that positively influence both of these areas, promoting health and wellness and increasing your efficiency. Factors that put you at risk for injury can also be reduced when your efficiency increases.

Workplace Environment

Enhancement of performance in the workplace is referred to as *ergonomics*. Occupational activities and postures can be improved by ergonomically arranged workstations. Ergonomic job analysis considers the demands required to perform your crucial work tasks. Observations, measurement of physical parameters, and interviews with you and your employer all provide information that can be used to enhance your work performance. In the field of industry, improved performance can help to create a safer workplace as well as to improve output. Adjustments that can create efficient and economical performance related to both production and fatigue include working position, speed of movement, and flow of movement. The doctor of chiropractic can assist you in designing an ergonomically safe and efficient work environment.

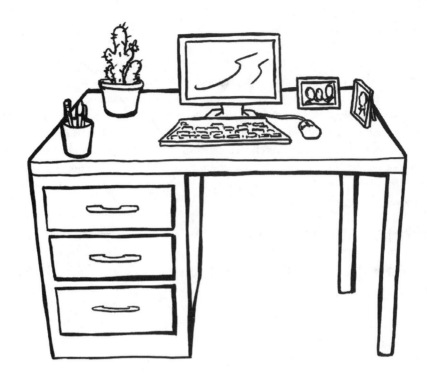

Identification of Workplace Risks

Pre-employment assessment by your chiropractor can identify if you are at high risk for injury associated with specific work activities. Pre-employment assessment does not provide employers with information that you should not be selected for high-risk tasks; rather, it identifies if you are at high risk should you seek employment that exposes you to certain stresses.[2] Assessment is based on your history, examination findings, and x-rays. Significant risk factors can then be evaluated relative to specific tasks. Education and training based on sound biomechanical principles can help you to adapt to job situations and enhance your performance. Factors that affect workplace efficiency include the following:

- Fitness
- Lifting and carrying
- Suitable seated posture
- Repetitive use

Avoidance of at-risk postures can prevent work-related injuries. A job that is modified to fit you as an individual can enhance your performance and increase your output.

FITNESS

Increasing your level of fitness can improve your performance and decrease your work-related risks (see Chapter 4). Regardless of whether you are involved in a sedentary occupation or in a job that requires heavy physical activity, being fit to work plays a significant part in your overall wellness. Work that leaves you unable to participate in enjoyable recreational activities at the end of the work period because of poor fitness levels severely decreases your quality of life. An individual assessment of your fitness level, with guidelines for the development of a realistic program for improved fitness, can enhance your work performance and can be provided by your doctor of chiropractic.

LIFTING AND CARRYING

Implementing the principles of proper body mechanics while limiting loads carried can improve performance and prevent injury. Accurate assessment of load limits appropriate for lifting can be calculated. You can be taught the proper techniques for lifting, pushing, pulling, and carrying by your doctor of chiropractic. Biomechanically health-promoting principles include the following:[3]

- *Keeping loads close to your torso:* The further away the load is from your center of gravity, the higher your risk of injury.
- *Not lifting loads from floor level:* The lower you lift from the floor, the greater the angle of forward bending and the higher the compression forces on your discs.
- *Avoiding ballistic or jerky motions:* Moving loads in a slow, planned manner minimizes any unexpected motions and prevents your loss of grip, slipping, and tripping.
- *Avoiding twisting and lateral bending when lifting:* If turning is necessary, pivoting on your feet avoids trunk rotation.
- *Minimizing carrying:* You can biomechanically lift more than you can carry; carrying should be kept to a minimum.
- *Avoiding bending forward with the legs straight while setting down a load:* You are less likely to sustain an injury to your back if you bend your knees while lowering a load.

SUITABLE SEATED POSTURE

Appropriate posture for prolonged sitting can also enhance work performance. Ergonomic factors that should be considered are seat height, seat angle, seat depth, cushioning, backrest angle, and armrests. Practicing adequate seated body mechanics is a valued self-care strategy that can contribute to your health and wellness.

Ergonomically designed seats ideally should include the following characteristics:[3]

- Seat height that allows you to place both feet firmly on the floor
- Seat angle that is individualized to suit you since seated postures can be stressful to the spine
- Seat depth that is adjustable if possible, with a compromise between your thigh support and your freedom of body movement
- A supportive backrest angle that partially relieves stress on the spine
- Cushioning that is relatively firm, with your body weight supported on the ischial tuberosities
- A backrest contour that supports your lumbar spine
- Armrests that provide support but do not extend so far as to interfere with arm movements
- Shock-absorbing seats that help to minimize vibratory stress that is detrimental to your spine

REPETITIVE USE

Stress from repetitive motion can compromise performance and lead to painful and disabling disorders. You should not perform work that requires repetitive movements for prolonged periods, and should intersperse such work with regular breaks. Alternating repetitive tasks with other jobs can minimize excessive muscular strain. *Repetitive strain injury* has become a pejorative term. It is also known as *cumulative trauma disorder*.

Prevention of a condition that some employers deny as work related is best dealt with by restricting tasks that involve repetitive hand movements to one to two hours at a time. Pacing with regular stretching can also be beneficial. Asymmetrical postures such as cradling a telephone between the neck and shoulders can result in myofascial pain and can be avoided with the use of a telephone headset.[4] An ergonomically designed computer station should be individualized to maximize efficiency. In addition to an ergonomically designed seat, an efficient and safe computer station should include the following:

- Placement of the source documents, the keyboard, and the monitor to minimize head movement

- Placement of the keyboard directly below the hands, with the elbows at about 90 degrees
- A rest for the forearms for long-term work
- Alignment of your body with the part of the keyboard used the most

Adaptation of your job through information and training can enhance your job performance through the use of sound ergonomic principles. Application of the rules administered by the Environmental Protection Agency and the Occupational Safety and Health Administration can be helpful in enhancing work performance and promoting health and wellness. Ergonomics can provide biomechanical solutions that reduce musculoskeletal stresses resulting from the environment, the task, the tools, and the workplace in general. Careful analysis of your activities and tasks, with appropriate recommendations from your doctor of chiropractic, can enhance your job-related performance. Ultimately, you are responsible for making the appropriate adjustments for efficiency, the minimization of fatigue, and maintenance of good working posture, but an ergonomically efficient and safe workplace must also be provided by your employer if your performance is to be optimized.

Recreational Activities

The importance of recreational activities to health promotion and wellness cannot be overstated. The joy of movement comes from the kinesthetic sensations of the rhythmic pattern of movement and the release of endorphins. Your self-image and overall well-being are both increased when your performance is improved.

Enhanced performance during recreational activities is commonly promoted through sports medicine. While some doctors of chiropractic specialize in sports medicine, the doctor of chiropractic who promotes health and wellness can also help you to improve the performance of your recreational activities. Assessment of your level of fitness is the first step in improving your performance. In addition to your regular health promotion examination, you will want an evaluation of your fitness level specific to your chosen activity. The specific activity examination should assess your risk of injury in addition to determining your baseline fitness level.

Preparticipation Evaluation

The preparticipation evaluation is performed with an eye toward injury prevention through assessment of risks associated with a specific activity. Common goals for the preparticipation evaluation include the following:[5]

- Determining your general health status
- Discovering any defects that limit participation
- Uncovering any conditions predisposing to injury
- Developing strategies for bringing you to your optimal level of performance
- Classifying you according to your individual qualifications
- Evaluating the size and level of maturation in younger patients
- Evaluating opportunities should you have a disability
- Modifying activities should you be an older individual

COMPONENTS OF THE PREPARTICIPATION EXAMINATION

Factors that should be considered when determining your suitability for a specific activity include the level of the activity and your previous experience. Factors that should be evaluated are outlined in Table 7.1.

Prerequisites of Efficient Movements

The prerequisites to efficient movement include physical, mental, and emotional factors, coordinated by the nervous system (Tables 7.2 to 7.5). There are general underlying functional characteristics common to all performance. Muscle strength, power, speed, endurance, and agility are elements that lay the foundation of all activities. In addition to a general level of fitness, the specific requirements of each sport vary according to the skills necessary to perform that activity. Each sport requires a variety of movement patterns.

Table 7.1 *Components of the Preparticipation Examination*

History of previous injuries, hospitalizations, and joint problems

History of heat-related illness or exercise-induced respiratory distress

Physical conditions such as heart murmurs, arrhythmias, or hypertension

Use of appliances, including contact lenses, glasses, and dental braces or bridges

Psychological appropriateness (contact sports or high-stress activities such as climbing or auto racing are not for everyone)

Strength imbalances that can contribute to injury

Flexibility imbalances around the hip and back

Adapted from the text of Fu FH, Stone DA. *Sports Injuries: Mechanisms, Prevention, Treatment.* Baltimore. Lippincott Williams & Wilkins; 1994.

Table 7.2 *Physical Prerequisites to Efficient Movements*

Endurance: organic, cardiorespiratory, muscular, and nervous

Flexibility: ligament, muscle, and joint

Strength: shoulder girdle, arm, wrist, hand, trunk abdominal, pelvic, leg, and foot

Muscular power: explosive strength and dynamic energy

Acuity of senses: visual, auditory, kinesthetic, tactile, and semicircular canals

Reaction time

Adapted from the text of Fu FH, Stone DA. *Sports Injuries: Mechanisms, Prevention, Treatment*. Baltimore. Lippincott Williams & Wilkins; 1994.

Table 7.3 *Mental Prerequisites to Efficient Movements*

Concentration

Perceiving quickly

Understanding the nature of the skill

Solving motor problems and quickly making adaptive decisions

Perceiving spatial relations

Judging moving objects

Applying rhythmic judgment: time, duration, stress, and intensity

Using kinesthetic memory: ability to remember past movement

Adapted from the text of Fu FH, Stone DA. *Sports Injuries: Mechanisms, Prevention, Treatment*. Baltimore. Lippincott Williams & Wilkins; 1994.

Table 7.4 *Emotional Prerequisites to Efficient Movement*

Desire to learn or perform a skill

A positive attitude toward performance

Self-control

Absence of disturbing emotional factors (fear of failure)

Adapted from the text of Fu FH, Stone DA. *Sports Injuries: Mechanisms, Prevention, Treatment*. Baltimore. Lippincott Williams & Wilkins; 1994.

Table 7.5 *Neurological Prerequisites to Efficient Movement*

Balance control: size of base, center of gravity, head orientation, alternation of arms and legs

Timing control: hand-eye and foot-eye coordination

Rhythm of movement of body parts: speed, sequence, and duration

Muscular control: voluntary movement and involuntary movement (steadiness)

Agility: ability to change direction quickly

Coordination: combining simple movements without unnecessary tension and in the proper sequence to make a smooth, complex movement

---

Adapted from the text of Fu FH, Stone DA. *Sports Injuries: Mechanisms, Prevention, Treatment*. Baltimore. Lippincott Williams & Wilkins; 1994.

Your body composition is closely related to your performance and susceptibility to injury. Your ratio of lean body tissue to fat tissue should be considered. The assessment of body composition involves the measurement of skinfold thickness.

Strength development needs to occur functionally, enhancing your selected performance characteristics. A specific strength training program can be designed to develop functional strength specific to your particular recreational activity. Appropriate warm-up before exercise and a warm-down after exercise reduce the risk of injuries. Stretching increases the flexibility of soft tissues around a joint and can enhance performance. "No pain, no gain" should be replaced with "train without pain."

The Importance of Play

The benefits of play include a release of tension that promotes pleasurable relaxation. The fun element relieves you from ordinary life by allowing you to abandon yourself in an activity that absorbs you intensely. Play lies outside morals and is neither good nor bad as long as the rules are followed. Your ability to participate efficiently in play can be more pleasurable with enhanced performance, but the freedom to participate in a voluntary activity should not be dependent on competition alone. Whether you compete with yourself or others, play should be an end in itself rather than a score in the end.

Emotionally meaningful and satisfying recreational activities are not only important to your health and wellness but can also delay the aging process. Learning efficient body mechanics early in life can enrich the later decades of life, but it is never too late to participate.

Guiding Principles of Performance Enhancement

The guiding principles of human performance that must be considered are as follows:

- All tissues of the body show a definite relationship between structure and function, with adaptations being made to functional demands that are both normal and pathological.
- Human motion occurs in accordance with general mechanical laws, applied to the structure and functioning of the neuromusculoskeletal system.
- The kinetic demands placed on you require complex adjustment through the application of mechanical laws to your individual structure and function.
- The quality of your daily life can be significantly improved through the enhancement of your performance in both work and recreational environments.

References

1. Scott MG. *Analysis of Human Movement*. 2nd ed. New York: Appleton Century Crofts; 1963.
2. Gatterman MI. *Chiropractic Management of Spine Related Disorders*. 2nd ed. Baltimore: Lippincott Williams & Wilkins; 2004:364.
3. Jamison JR. *Health Promotion for Chiropractic Practice*. Gaithersburg, MD: Aspen; 1991:167–172.
4. Rachlin ES, Rachlin IS. *Myofascial Pain and Fibromyalgia: Trigger Point Management*. 2nd ed. St. Louis: Mosby; 2002.
5. Fu FH, Stone DA. *Sports Injuries: Mechanisms, Prevention, Treatment*. Baltimore: Lippincott Williams & Wilkins; 1994.

Chapter 8

Finding Your Wellness Doctor of Chiropractic

The doctor of the future will give no medicines, but will interest his patients in the care of the human frame, in diet, and in the causes of disease.

Thomas Edison

I t is important that you find a patient-centered doctor of chiropractic who can provide you with health promotion and wellness care. A patient-centered approach emphasizes communication, partnership, and health promotion.[1]

- The doctor must be approachable, friendly, and communicate with you in language that you understand.

- As you work with your doctor, a partnership develops in the patient/doctor relationship that is based on mutual discussion.

- Health promotion that focuses on relating to the whole person, not a disease or disorder of your body part, is central to wellness care.

Access to patient-centered practitioners who promote health and wellness is based on availability and appropriateness, preferences, and timeliness.[2]

Availability and Appropriateness

How do I find a health promotion and wellness doctor of chiropractic in my area? The answer to this question is finding a health promotion and wellness practitioner in your area. Northwestern Health Sciences University offers a certificate program in Integrative Health and Wellness. Graduates of this program understand the importance of health promotion and wellness and have the ability to apply their knowledge in this area. They must demonstrate competence, compassion, and care in the service of patients from all cultural and spiritual backgrounds. They must understand the importance of actively managing and maintaining one's own health and wellness, including the integration of body, mind, and spirit. Courses taken in the clinical track include the following:

- Principles of Integrative Health, Wellness, and Practice
- Healing, Health, and Culture
- Health and Wellness Counseling
- Exercise and Clinical Nutrition

Information on graduates of this program is available from the university (see Appendix B).

A second source for finding health promotion and wellness doctors is the American Chiropractic Association. You want to look for practitioners who are trained to counsel patients on healthy habits and lifestyle and who have developed skills and strategies for working with patients in a partnership for shared decision making.

Health Promotion and Wellness practitioners emphasize the following:

- Wellness promotion and counseling for lifestyle modification
- Nutrition and essentials for healthy eating
- Posture and spinal health, physical activity and exercise, and mental fitness
- Occupational health and work safety

Information on Certified Health Promotion and Wellness practitioners in your area is available from the American Chiropractic Association (see Appendix B).

Appropriateness involves obtaining the proper level of care. It is important that the health promotion and wellness practitioner has the knowledge to help you filter and interpret appropriate information specific to you. An individual approach to your healthcare needs is a primary characteristic of patient-centered care.

Preference

Your preferences are based on your experiences and the recommendations of others. A key factor in your satisfaction with any healthcare practitioner is your relationship with your healthcare provider. A doctor of chiropractic who is willing to work with you as a partner in making decisions affecting your health and wellness is essential. Finding a suitable doctor of chiropractic whose practice includes health promotion and wellness counseling includes physical proximity and ease of access. Most importantly, one who respects your preferences is in your best interest.

Timeliness

Timeliness concerns receiving care and counseling when desired. Your readiness to make lifestyle changes must adhere to your time schedule. It is futile to receive information and instruction on changes toward healthier habits if you are not ready to act on these changes. The doctor of chiropractic can promote your health and wellness by providing the necessary information, but the ultimate factor in your success is you.

Your Health Promotion and Wellness Plan

Your plan of action to achieve improved health and wellness includes defining your goals, your motivation, a plan to follow, a means of measuring your progress, and rewards for success.

- Defining your goals must be based on a realistic assessment of your current health status. Your doctor of chiropractic can make this assessment using a variety of screening tools in addition to a thorough physical examination.
- Your motivation to follow your plan of action will be based on your personal needs and desires. You must ask yourself why your goals are important to you. For example, you may wish to have more energy, be able to participate more fully in physical activity, and enjoy an improved sense of well-being.
- Your action plan outlines clearly the steps to follow in your journey to wellness. It may include weight loss or weight gain. You must clearly recognize what has tripped you up in the past and create a plan to avoid such pitfalls.
- Keeping track of your progress may include keeping a journal or diary. Recognizing milestones allows you to experience success and can further your motivation to continue your plan.
- Celebrating success is an important part of your increased wellness. Increased self-esteem has its own rewards, as does an improvement in your sense of well-being. Additional rewards may include a long-overdue vacation or something as simple as buying a book you want or seeking out entertainment that you enjoy.[3]

Mind-set for a New Model

Doctors of chiropractic who practice health promotion and wellness care follow a model very different from the prevailing healthcare model. Rather than focusing on diseases of body parts, they view the individual as a whole. Emphasis is placed on optimizing function through maintenance of a healthy lifestyle. Assessment of realistic personal health risks is tailored to you as an individual. Doctors of chiropractic have an important role to play in coaching you to undertake appropriate and effective lifestyle changes that promote health and wellness. Wellness is a multidimensional concept that includes physical, psychological, social, and spiritual aspects. It is important to sever the shackles of the disease-based model and embrace a more holistic paradigm that can make profound changes in your health and well-being.

References

1. Little P, Everitt H, Williamson I, Warner G, Moore M, Gould C, Ferrier K, Payne S. Preferences of patients for patient centered approach to consultation in primary care: observational study. *BMJ*. 2001;322:1–7.

2. Berry L, Seiders K, Wilder S. Innovations in access to care: a patient centered approach. *Ann Intern Med*. 2003;139:568–574.

3. Jamison JR. *Maintaining Health in Primary Care: Guidelines for Wellness in the 21st Century*. St. Louis: Churchill Livingstone; 2001.

Straighten Up America: Fitness Fun for Everyone

Ron Kirk

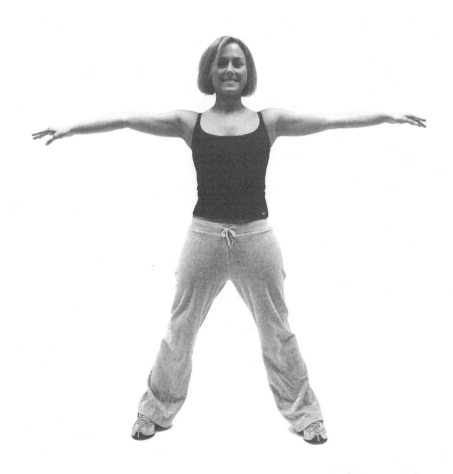

A Short History and Introduction to Straighten Up

S pearheaded by the chiropractic profession, Straighten Up is a bold and in-novative health initiative designed to empower people in an improved quality of life and healthy lifestyle.

The vision driving Straighten Up is very simple. We envision a time when everyone will take two or three minutes every day to care for their spinal health, just as they care for their dental health. The need for spinal health promotion is very great, as evidenced by the many billions of dollars spent each year related to spinal disability. Yet before Straighten Up, there had not been a short, simple, engaging spinal exercise program designed to promote the public's spinal health.

To address this problem in the summer of 2004, a five-person expert seed panel and a multidisciplinary Delphi review panel of approximately 100 health-care clinicians, professional association leaders, college presidents, researchers, and health promotion experts began shaping and testing a spinal exercise module known as Straighten Up America. A free, public service program, Straighten Up is packed into three minutes of fun, engaging, healthful activities. Equally useful as an ergonomic break, exercise warm-up, or cool-down, Straighten Up is de-signed to get people of all ages and ethnicity up and moving, while they improve their posture and spinal health. The program also includes a short set of healthy lifestyle recommendations congruent with the goals and objectives of national and international physical activity and health promotion initiatives.

Though still in its infancy as a health initiative, Straighten Up has garnered a number of accolades from health and fitness leaders, including Lee Haney, past chairman of the U.S. President's Council on Physical Fitness and Sports. He de-scribes the program as "awesome," with "vision and much promise." In January 2005, Tommy Thompson, then U.S. Secretary of Health and Human Services, "commended" the individuals who developed Straighten Up for their "leadership in the field of spinal health."

Results from tests of the program are very promising. After five weeks of daily practice of Straighten Up exercises, 83% of study participants reported that they had improved their posture. Seventy-eight percent reported that they had strengthened their core muscles. Eighty percent reported that they sat and stood more upright and that their backs were more comfortable.

Participants in our initial study ranged from college students to individuals in their eighties. Young children that we have taught also love Straighten Up and are practicing it enthusiastically. We hope that children around the world will prac-tice these beneficial spinal health habits. Dr. Jose Carlos Martines, the director of the Child and Adolescent Health and Development Cluster of the World Health

Organization, shares this hope and helped to shape the program as a Delphi panel member. We are currently creating multiple language translations of Straighten Up for global implementation and habituation.

To date, Straighten Up has received enthusiastic reviews wherever it has been presented. Some of these venues were as follows:

- The U.S. House of Representatives Wellness Center
- The U.S. Bone and Joint Decade Meeting at the National Institutes of Health
- The American Public Health Association Annual Meeting
- The World Federation of Chiropractic/Foundation for Chiropractic Education Research Conference in Sydney, Australia
- The Chiropractic Coalition Summit
- The Association of Chiropractic Colleges/Research Agenda Annual Conference
- The Congress of Chiropractic State Associations Annual Convention

For more information regarding Straighten Up, you may inquire at www.life.edu under the header "Chiropractic and Wellness" or at www.cocsa.org.

After you have consulted with your doctor of chiropractic, if you do not have conditions limiting shoulder and arm motion, we suggest beginning to practice Straighten Up by first performing the Posture Pod regularly. The Posture Pod provides an excellent ergonomic break or warm-up or cool-down for other forms of exercise. It takes only about 30 to 40 seconds to perform. Once you have mastered the Posture Pod, you may begin practicing the full Straighten Up program for postural improvement and core stabilization. We recommend performing Straighten Up in concert with the exercise recommendations of your chiropractor or other healthcare practitioner. Always check with your doctor before beginning an activity-based program to make sure the activities are appropriate for you.

Straighten Up America: Healthy Child and Adult Version

Key Features

1. Three minutes long for quick daily conditioning
2. Health enhancing and fun

3. Simple enough for almost anyone
4. No special equipment needed
5. Helps you look and feel better
6. Easy and convenient

Program Goals

1. To improve posture and function
2. To stabilize core musculature
3. To enhance spinal and neurological health
4. To prevent spinal subluxations

Basic Rules

1. Think positively. Enjoy the moment. This is serious fun.
2. Straighten up. Stand tall with a confident "inner winner" posture (ears, shoulders, hips, knees, and ankles in an approximately straight line).
3. Breathe calmly, deeply, and slowly from your stomach region.
4. Move smoothly. Do not jerk or bounce.

Notice

Check with your doctor or chiropractic or other healthcare practitioner before beginning Straighten Up to make sure the exercises are appropriate for you and your specific needs. If you experience recurring, sharp or shooting pain, stop and report back to your doctor. You may need to modify the exercises.

Four Segments of Straighten Up

1. Spine Tuning Warm-Up (Tilting Star, Twirling Star, Twisting Star)
2. Postural Pod (Trap Openers, the Eagle, the Hummingbird, the Butterfly)
3. Balancing the Core (Tightrope)
4. Wrapping It Up (Banging the Gong, Extending the Sword, Shaking It Loose)

"Inner Winner" Posture

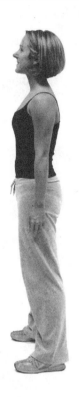

1. Straighten up. Stand tall with a confident "inner winner" posture (ears, shoulders, hips, knees, and ankles in an approximately straight line).

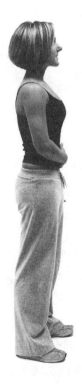

2. Pull your belly button in toward your spine.

Spine Tuning Warm-up Preview

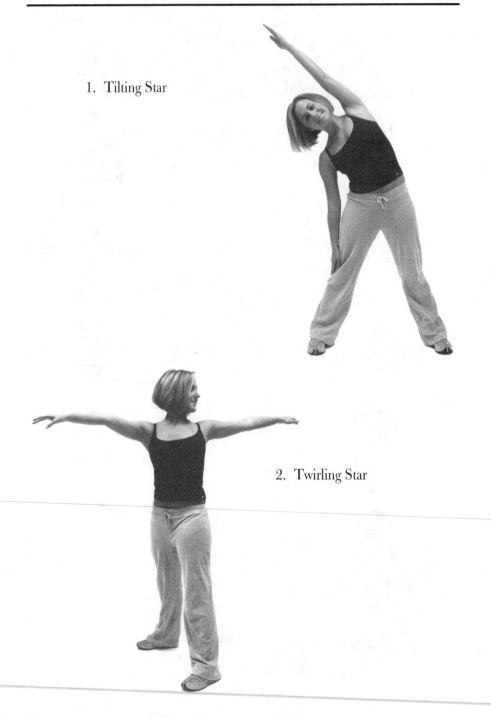

1. Tilting Star

2. Twirling Star

3. Twisting Star

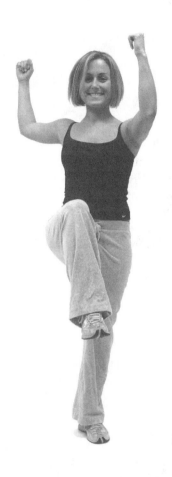

Tilting Star

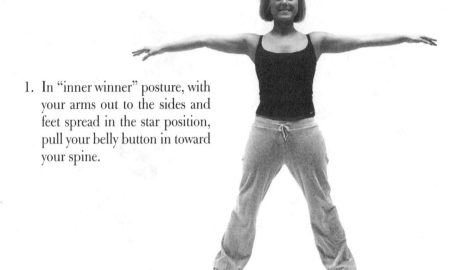

1. In "inner winner" posture, with your arms out to the sides and feet spread in the star position, pull your belly button in toward your spine.

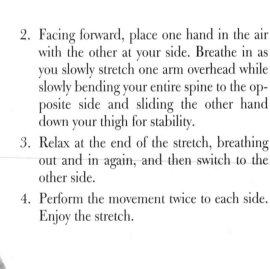

2. Facing forward, place one hand in the air with the other at your side. Breathe in as you slowly stretch one arm overhead while slowly bending your entire spine to the opposite side and sliding the other hand down your thigh for stability.

3. Relax at the end of the stretch, breathing out and in again, and then switch to the other side.

4. Perform the movement twice to each side. Enjoy the stretch.

Twirling Star

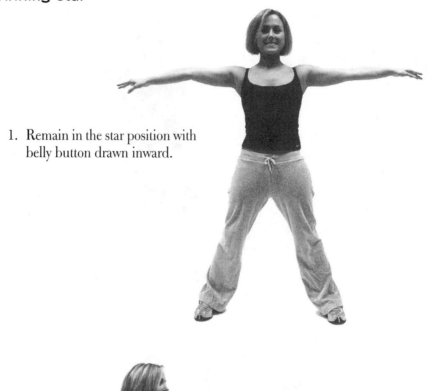

1. Remain in the star position with belly button drawn inward.

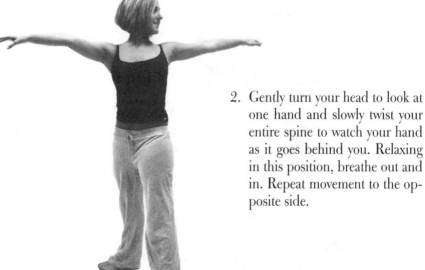

2. Gently turn your head to look at one hand and slowly twist your entire spine to watch your hand as it goes behind you. Relaxing in this position, breathe out and in. Repeat movement to the opposite side.

Twisting Star

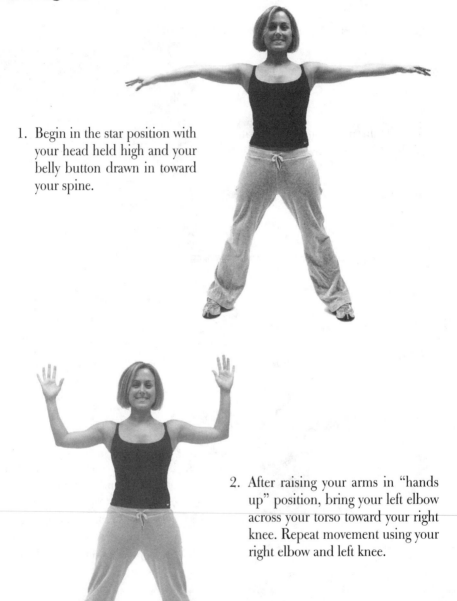

1. Begin in the star position with your head held high and your belly button drawn in toward your spine.

2. After raising your arms in "hands up" position, bring your left elbow across your torso toward your right knee. Repeat movement using your right elbow and left knee.

3. Remain upright as you continue to alternate for 15 seconds. Breathe freely. Enjoy.

4. Individuals with balance disorders should use caution if attempting this exercise.

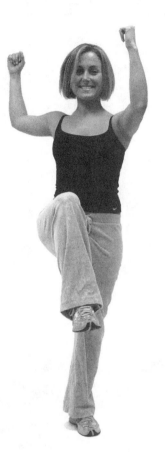

Posture Pod Preview

1. Trap Openers

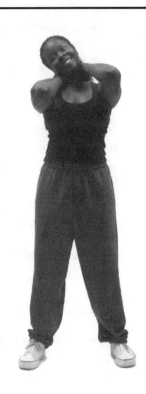

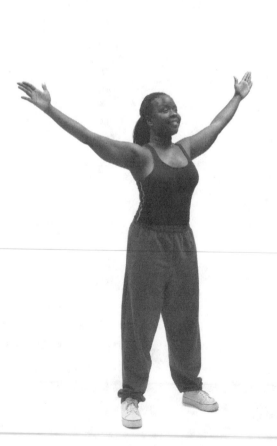

2. The Eagle

3. The Hummingbird

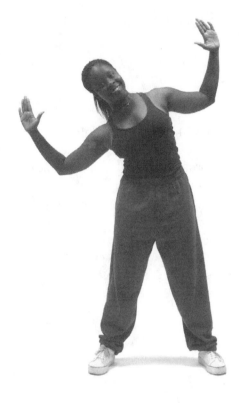

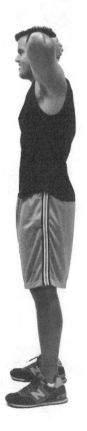

4. The Butterfly

Trap Openers

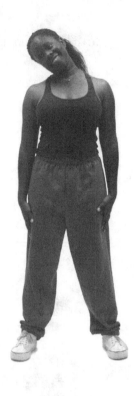

1. Breathe deeply and calmly, relaxing your stomach region. Let your head hang loosely forward and gently roll from one side to the other.

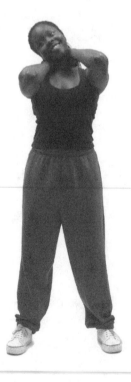

2. Using your fingers, slowly massage the area just below the back of your head. Move down to the base of your neck.

3. Then relax your shoulders and slowly roll them backwards and forwards. Enjoy for 15 seconds.

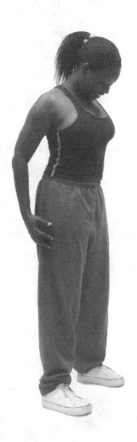

The Eagle and the Hummingbird

1. In "inner winner" posture, pull your belly button in toward your spine. To begin the Eagle, bring your arms out to the sides and gently draw your shoulder blades together. Breathe in as you slowly raise your arms, touching your hands together above your head. Slowly lower your arms to your sides as you breathe out. Perform movement three times.

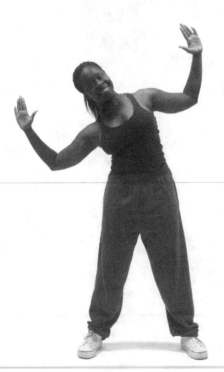

2. Next make small backward circles with your hands and arms, swaying from side to side in the Hummingbird. Enjoy for 10 seconds.

The Butterfly

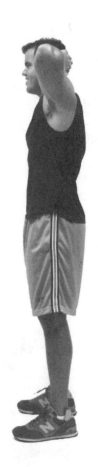

1. Place your hands behind your head and gently draw your elbows backward. Slowly and gently press your head backward and resist with your hands for a count of two and release. Breathe freely. Perform three times.

2. Gently massage the back of your neck and head as you relax your stomach region with slow, easy breathing.

Balancing the Core with the Tightrope

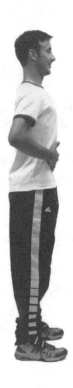

1. Stand in "inner winner" position with your head held high. Contract your stomach muscles to pull your belly button in toward your spine.

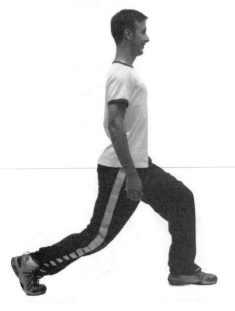

2. Maintaining this posture, take a step forward as if on a tightrope. Make sure your knee is over your ankle and not over your toes. Allow the heel of your back foot to lift. Balance in this position for 20 seconds. Repeat on the opposite side. When finished, shake your legs and feet to relax them.

Wrapping It Up Preview

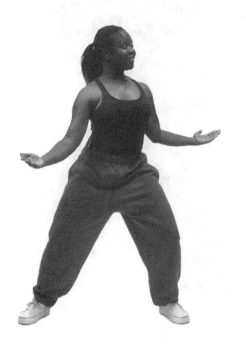

1. Banging the Gong

2. Extending the Sword

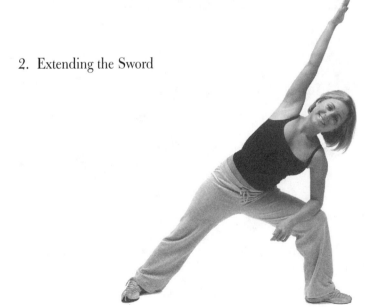

3. Shaking It Loose

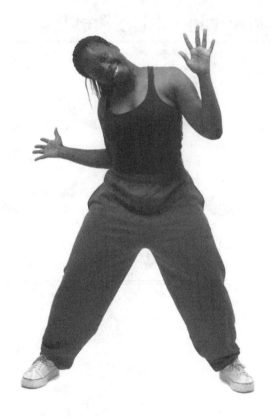

Banging the Gong

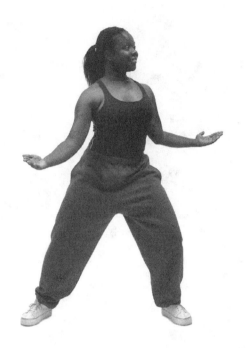

1. Standing tall in "inner winner" posture with your feet wider than your shoulders, pull your belly button in toward your spine. Then gently rotate your trunk from side to side. Easy does it.

2. Let your arms flop loosely as you shift your weight from knee to knee.

3. Swing gently from side to side. Breathe calmly and deeply. Enjoy the movement for 15 seconds.

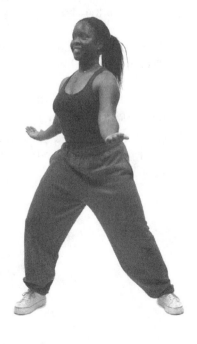

Extending the Sword

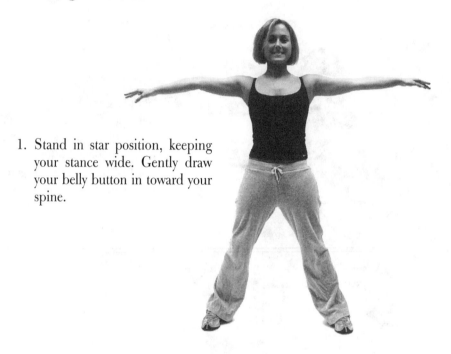

1. Stand in star position, keeping your stance wide. Gently draw your belly button in toward your spine.

2. Turn your foot outward as you shift your weight to one side. Feel the groin area gently stretching. Place your knee over your ankle and your elbow behind your knee as you extend your arm, torso, and ribs. Easy does it.

3. Older adults should place their hand on their knee. Stretch for 10 seconds on each side.

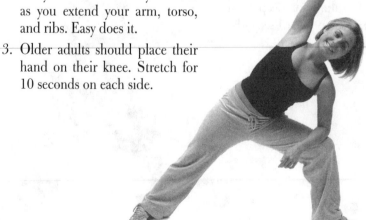

Shaking it Loose

1. Shake limbs loosely for 15 seconds.

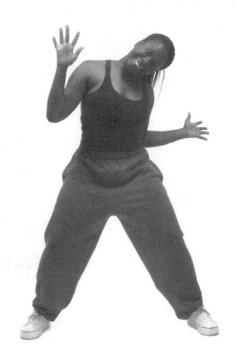

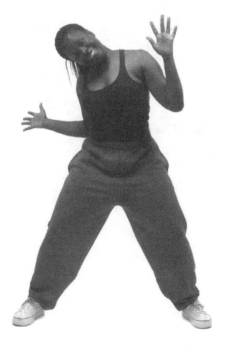

2. This one is pure fun.
3. We are done!

Getting Started with Straighten Up America

1. Straighten Up America is intended to be incorporated in a healthy lifestyle of prudent active living. Consistent healthy choices and healthful habits form the bedrock of a healthy life. Our hope is that you make Straighten Up a daily part of a vibrant empowering lifestyle for the whole family.

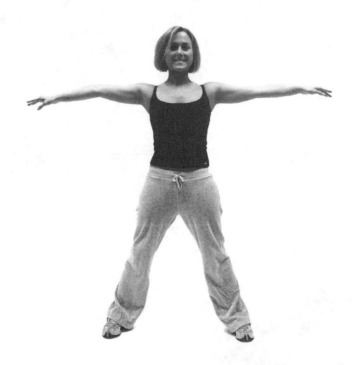

2. This version of Straighten Up is designed for healthy children and adults to practice daily, like brushing your teeth.
3. Consult with your doctor of chiropractic or other healthcare provider before practicing this module, especially if you have spinal disabilities or other disorders that limit movement.

Straighten Up Lifestyle Choices

1. *Choose to Improve.* You are worth it. Maintain a positive perspective. Take small steps at first, set specific measurable health goals, and achieve them. Celebrate your health successes, learn from temporary setbacks, and move on. Choose to see life as an adventure. Keep learning for a lifetime.

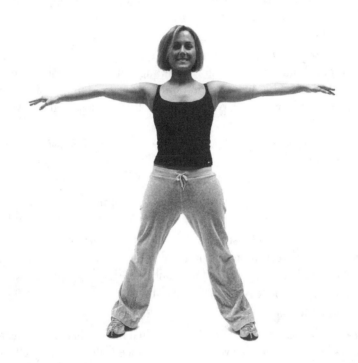

2. *Choose to enjoy healthy, invigorating activity at least 30 minutes daily when possible.* Begin slowly, making gradual improvements. Keep an activity log or calendar. If you buy a pedometer, you can count or track your steps. Choosing active hobbies will add variety and spice to your life. Exercise for flexibility, balance, strength, and endurance. Perform Straighten Up daily to improve your posture and strengthen your core muscles.

3. *Choose to live tobacco free for your personal health and for your loved ones.* Tobacco has detrimental effects on your nervous system and skeletal structures, as well as on your heart and lungs.

4. *Choose healthy foods.* Eat naturally. Enjoy whole grain breads and cereals. Choose several daily helpings of fresh fruit and vegetables rich in anti-oxidants and phytonutrients. Calcium- and magnesium-rich foods help to build strong spinal columns. Avoid saturated and *trans* fats found in fast, fried foods. Instead, eat more omega-3 fats from flax products and small ocean fish for healthy spine joints. Choose high-quality protein foods. Avoid refined sweets, such as sodas and candy. When supplementing your diet with vitamins and minerals, make quality choices. Try to eat in a re-laxed atmosphere.

5. *Choose good posture while sitting, standing, or lifting.* Hold your head high; keep your shoulders back. Lift by bending your legs with objects held close to your torso. This helps to prevent injury. Take frequent mini breaks. Segments of Straighten Up work well for this purpose. Change work posi-tions often.

6. *Choose a balanced supportive book bag or backpack for school, work, or recre-ation.* Carry less weight at one time. Use a bag with broad, padded straps se-curely positioned on both shoulders.

7. *Choose a comfortable supportive mattress.* For optimal spinal health, sleep on your side or on your back, not face down. Plan for sufficient restful sleep.

8. *Choose to be quiet.* The stress of life affects your health and your posture. Take time for relaxation and renewal. Practice thankfulness and positive thinking. Reflect, pray, or meditate daily. Read uplifting writings.

9. *Choose to serve others.* Volunteerism and service enhance the quality of our lives and our relationships.

10. *Choose to be kind to your spine.* Regular spinal health checkups, care, and ex-ercises help to ensure that your spine is balanced, aligned, and well adjusted. A healthy spine and nervous system add balance and harmony to life.

Resources

ACA Wellness Certification Program
American Chiropractic Association
1701 Clarendon Boulevard
Arlington, Virginia 22209
Phone: 1-800-986-4636

Integrative Health and Wellness
Northwestern Health Sciences University
2501 West 84th Street
Minneapolis, Minnesota 55431
Phone: 1-952-888-4777

Federation of Chiropractic Licensing Boards
5101 West 10th Street, Suite 101
Greeley, Colorado 80634
Phone: 1-970-356-3500

Index